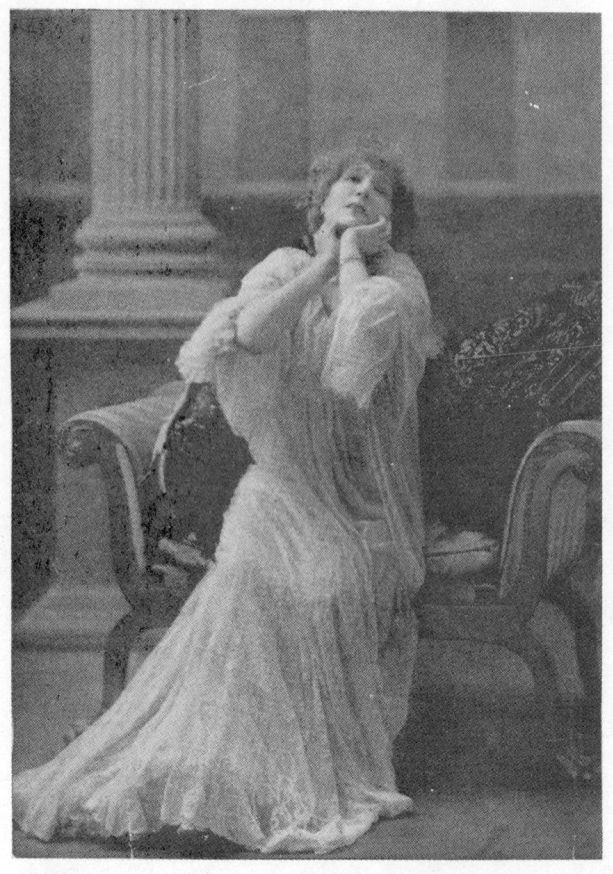

SARAH BERNHARDT 1905
In the part of Adrienne Lecouvreur in the play of that name written by herself. (By permission of D. & D. Downey.)

SARAH BERNHARDT

BY
MAURICE BARING

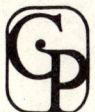

GREENWOOD PRESS, PUBLISHERS
WESTPORT, CONNECTICUT

252632

Copyright © 1934 by D. Appleton-Century Company, Inc.

Originally published in 1934
by Appleton-Century Company, Inc.

Reprinted from a copy in the collections
of the Brooklyn Public Library

First Greenwood Reprinting 1970

Library of Congress Catalogue Card Number 70-98809

SBN 8371-3018-2

PRINTED IN UNITED STATES OF AMERICA

NOTE

THE authorities I have consulted in writing this short book are all mentioned in the text. I have to thank M. Pierre Sardou, M. Couët, keeper of the archives at the Théâtre Français, M. Louis Verneuil, and M. C. du Bousquet for their valuable assistance, and Mr. Edward Marsh for reading the proofs.

M. B.

CHAPTER I

To write the life of Sarah Bernhardt it would require another Sarah Bernhardt: that is to say, someone who could do in biography what she could do in acting. Whether such a person exists at the present moment, I do not know; all I know is that I am not that person.

All that I shall attempt will be a few sidelights, based to a certain extent upon what I have heard and read, and to a greater extent on what I have seen myself.

When Sarah Bernhardt died, on 26th March 1923, a Frenchman in a biographical sketch of her said that her life was shot with thunder and lightning: it was a whirlwind of dates, titles, gleaming swords, fireworks, poets and prose-writers, men of genius and clever men, garlands, smiles, prayers and tears. A great clamour arises from it: applause, sobs, whistling trains, steamers screaming in the fog; a kaleidoscope of all countries; a babel of all tongues; shouts of enthusiasm, ejaculations of worship, cries of passion. Nobody could tell of all this in a short book.

All I shall attempt to do is to give a few glimpses of the gigantic and whirling peep-show, and to point out a few facets of the many-coloured kaleidoscope.

Henry James, in a novel, *The Tragic Muse,* chose as his subject the actress: *The* Actress, belonging to no time and to no country; international, bi-lingual, preferably Jewish, or with a streak of Jewish blood. He aimed at drawing the character and tracing the career of The Great Actress, and he partially succeeded. In an exaggerated foreshortening he gave the reader a hint of the essence of actors of genius, and of the kind of thing that happens to them.

In writing of his heroine he says: 'Her character was simply to hold you by the particular spell; any other—the good-nature of home, the relation to her mother, her friends, her lovers, her debts, the practice of virtues or industries or vices—was not worth speaking of. They were the fictions and shows; the representation was the deep substance.'

SARAH BERNHARDT

These words apply to the life of Sarah Bernhardt. She was an actress; her life was spent upon the boards acting, and in rehearsing when she was not acting: that was all that counted. All the rest: her voyages round and round the world, up and down the provinces of every country; her bankruptcies, her fortunes, her lovers, her marriage, her passions, her escapes and escapades on earth, air, fire and water, in ships, in mines, on glaciers, in balloons—these were like her sculpture, her painting, her playwriting . . . they did not count: they were but fiction and shows, side-shows, side-issues: utterly unimportant.

Her performance on the boards, her rehearsals: these were the deep substance.

For this reason I am going to make no attempt to tell the story of Sarah Bernhardt's private life. It does not matter, for it did not really exist.

What matters is her public life, which began in a convent She was born at Paris, at No. 265 Rue St. Honoré, on the 22nd October 1844. She was the daughter of well-to-do parents. We hear little of her father. He died young, and she never knew him. She does not mention him in her *Memoirs.* Her mother was Dutch. She describes her like this:

'My mother was a Jewess, and Dutch. She was fair-haired, small, soft and rounded (*boulotte*),[1] with a long figure and short legs, but a pretty face and wonderful blue eyes, and the head of the *Madonna della Seggiola.*'

Sarah Bernhardt's grandmother was one of eighteen; her mother bore fourteen children; Sarah was the eleventh. Sarah's mother was not only beautiful, but famous for her beauty. She was fond of travel. Sarah's childhood was managed by her uncle, who later became a Carthusian monk, and by her godfather, rather than by her mother. She was after a time especially looked after by a Madame Guérard, a friend of her mother, who, to the end of her life, never left Sarah.

Sarah was put in charge of a nurse in Brittany, and then under that of a Parisian *concierge,* while her mother galloped over Europe. Finally, her mother having settled at Paris, Sarah was sent to a school, and then to the convent of Grand-Champ at Versailles, of the Order of the Augustines. At this convent she was baptized.

[1] Untranslatable.

SARAH BERNHARDT

She was twelve years old, frail of health, 'tameless, swift and proud.' It was at the convent that she appeared for the first time in public. She acted in a religious play called *Tobit*, which was given in honour of the visit of the Cardinal Archbishop of Paris, Monseigneur Sigour. Sarah played the part of the Angel Raphael, and apparently she played it very well.

She spent two happy years at the convent, not without storms; and when they came to an end she had only one wish, to come back, no longer as a pupil but as a teacher. She was convinced that she had a vocation for the religious life. Her godfather said she must wait two years.

From the accounts she has left us of her childhood in her *Memoirs*, we see clearly that the child was the mother of the woman; there are in her own account of her early adventures, enthusiasms, hopes and fears, quarrels and escapades, sudden fits of temper and of tears, the same ungovernable impulses, the same outbursts of generosity and contractions of jealousy and explosions of fury, which she says herself in her *Memoirs* were more like fits of madness than of anger: the same sudden brain-storms, and paroxysms of panic and remorse; and at the back of all this, and throughout all this, the same indomitable fighting spirit, the same unconquerable will, and the determination to have her own way and to go her own way at all costs and in spite of all opposition, that distinguished her conduct and her career to the end of her life. She chose as a girl the untranslatable motto, *'Quand même'* (Withal and in spite of all); she acted up to her motto until the day of her death. It was when she was fourteen and a half that her relations, her mother, uncle and godfather, and the Duc de Morny, a friend of the family (and especially of her mother), met in conclave, the *conseil de famille,* to decide the future of Sarah Bernhardt. Her father had died, leaving her a marriage-portion of a hundred thousand francs, which she was not to receive until the day of her marriage. Her mother had only an annuity, and, as Sarah would not hear of marriage, the only alternative seemed to be to find for her a career which should make her independent. Sarah said she wanted to go back to the convent and become a nun; the discussion became heated, and Sarah pleaded her cause with so much vehemence and passion that the Duc de Morny, witnessing the scene, and his prophetic soul perhaps scenting dramatic talent, said: 'You ought to send that girl to the Conservatoire' (the famous school of dramatic art where pupils who wish to enter the Comédie Française are trained).

'She is far too thin to be an actress,' said her godfather; and Sarah continued in a torrent of words to vow that nothing would make her become an actress.

That night they took her to the Théâtre Français, and she sat through a performance of *Britannicus* in floods of tears, tears of homesickness for her convent, paying no attention to the play or to the actors; little dreaming, as she says in her *Memoirs*, that the curtain of that stage, which she saw go up for the first time, was destined to be the curtain of her life.

It was settled that she was to enter the Conservatoire, and for the first time in her life she began to read books: poetry and plays. I do not think she ever read anything else except poetry and plays all her life: nothing, that is, that was not grist to the mill of her art; and she soon knew the *Fables* of La Fontaine by heart. But, in order to enter the Conservatoire, it is necessary to pass an examination. The pupils have to act a scene or to recite a speech, and are only received if they satisfy the board of examiners. Sarah learned a scene from one of Molière's plays; but when the day of the examination came, and the moment for her to choose a fellow pupil from among the boy candidates to play the scene with her, she refused point-blank to act with any of them: saying that she did not know them.

'Then what will you say?' asked the stage manager, who was in charge of these recitations.

'A fable,' she answered, and the stage manager laughed as he put down on the list *Les Deux Pigeons,* by La Fontaine.

She got up on to the platform, where there was a jury of actors and actresses under the presidency of Monsieur Auber, the Director of the Conservatoire. No sooner had she spoken the opening lines of the fable,

> Deux Pigeons s'aimaient d'amour tendre:
> L'un d'eux s'ennuyant au logis . . .

than at least one member of the jury was struck by the undefinable thrill of being in the presence of something new, something *different,*

SARAH BERNHARDT

something rare. After two false starts and a certain amount of interruption, Sarah's matchless voice for the first of many thousand times imposed silence on a hardened, jaded and sceptical audience. There was no need for her to say the fable to the end; the President rang his bell, and as she walked down the steps, she was told that she had been admitted into the Conservatoire. The recitation of the first few lines of that fable contained as in a microcosm the whole of Sarah Bernhardt's career. She was never to say or to do anything better. No one else was ever to say anything so well.

Later on, in Scribe and Legouvé's play, *Adrienne Lecouvreur,* Sarah used to recite these same lines. Those who heard her say them knew that for the perfect utterance of beautiful words this was the Pillar of Hercules of mortal achievement: they had listened to the loveliest accents that had ever been spoken by mortal lips.

Her life was now revolutionised. Her determination, and with it her career, were fixed. She determined to be someone. She told me once herself that even in those early days she had felt no real attraction for the stage. As a child she had wanted to be a nun, and later on an artist—a painter or a sculptor; but, if she was to be an actress, well, she would be the first and the best. It was at this moment that this determination, perhaps unconsciously, but surely nevertheless, was crystallised.

Nothing went smoothly at first. In the first *concours* of the Conservatoire she obtained a second prize in tragedy and a 'first *accessit* in comedy, and the next year at the *concours* she obtained nothing in tragedy and the second prize in comedy. She tells in her *Memoirs* characteristic and amusing stories about these competitions: how, before the second *concours*, the hairdresser insisted on curling her hair (which to the end of her life she never 'did,' save by ruffling it and putting a pin through it) into tightly-pomaded curls; and how the passion and rage and tears with which she undid them, or tried to, leaving her with swollen eyes and a snuffling voice, prevented her from doing her best, or indeed from acting at all, in one of the scenes in which she had to appear. Nevertheless, in spite of these half-successes, she was admitted into the Comédie Française. She made her first appearance on the 11th August 1862, in Racine's *Iphigénie*. Sarcey, the dramatic critic, who devoted his whole life to the French stage, going to a play every night of his life and sitting through every play from the beginning to the end, and following the career of every actor or actress of note with meticulous conscientiousness until his death, wrote that her appearance was agreeable, that she held herself well, and said her words perfectly distinctly. That was all there was to say at present. He was less satisfied with her two following appearances (in Molière), and then, after quarrelling with one of the company, and after boxing the ears of an older actress, Madame Natalie, and a disappointment over a part which was first given to and then taken away from her, she sent in her resignation and left the Comédie Française, to which she was not to return for twelve years.

She was then engaged at the Gymnase, but she had no sooner acted in one or two parts than she felt an irrepressible desire to go to Spain. She left suddenly, and spent a fortnight there. Sardou relates afterwards that he happened to be in the manager's office at the Gymnase when the manager, Montigny, received Sarah's letter saying she had started for Spain. Recognising her handwriting, Montigny said: 'Oh, it's from that child.'

'Is she ill?' asked Sardou.

'No,' said the bearer of the letter. 'She has gone to Spain.'

'She can go to the devil,' said the manager.

'She must be rather fun,' said Sardou.

'Yes, but not for managers,' said Montigny.

When she came back from Spain she was engaged at the Porte Saint-Martin, where she acted in pantomime, and even sang, although she was musically tone-deaf; and, after more struggles and vicissitudes, she was engaged at the Odéon. Here, again, she made another first appearance which attracted no attention. But she worked hard, and played many parts, and notice and success came to her at last in the performance of Racine's *Athalie,* where she was allowed, since the choruses were going wrong when they were sung, to speak the stanzas; and here again her voice not only silenced criticism but came as a revelation. She soon became the favourite of the students in the gallery. But the first success that made her known to a larger public, and that brought her any meed of real fame, was her playing in a play in verse by a then unknown poet, François Coppée, called *Le Passant* (1869). The first performance of this lovely little play was a triumph. It ran for over a hundred nights to crowded houses, and the Emperor Napoleon III. had it performed at the Tuileries.

Sarah Bernhardt was now more than the favourite, she was the queen and the idol of the students on the other side of the river. It is interesting to note how prolonged was this seemingly uneventful prologue to her startling career: a scarcely noticed début at the Français; then twelve years of varied apprenticeship, ranging from comedy and melodrama to pantomime, before she again re-enters its portals as an actress who really counted: and even then she was far from fame. How slow real life is compared to fiction! How exaggerated is the foreshortening of the novelist! When an artist, such as Henry James, uses the career of a great artist as a theme of fiction in *The Tragic Muse,* he is obliged for the conduct of the story to foreshorten the apprenticeship, and to telescope eleven years into a period of two. He was later conscious himself of this fault in his book, and noted it in the

SARAH BERNHARDT

Preface. Sarah Bernhardt never woke up and found herself famous. Her fame was built up gradually, brick by brick, like a fantastic tower, which startled the world at every stage of its elevation, and was never finished. She was always learning: and she was working for the cinematograph when she died.

CHAPTER II

NOT long after the production of *Le Passant*, Sarah Bernhardt experienced her first serious financial crisis, which was caused by a fire in her Paris apartment, that broke out one night after dinner, and destroyed everything she possessed. Then came the Franco-Prussian War, during which she worked in an ambulance at the Odéon throughout the bombardment. She had many adventures, in France, and even, after the armistice, in Germany; for she went to Homburg to fetch her family in 1871.

The Odéon reopened its doors in January 1871. Sarah Bernhardt enjoyed a great success in a one-act play by André Theuriet, *Jean-Marie* (it has the same plot as *Enoch Arden*), which long afterwards she played to Queen Victoria at Nice.

Her reputation was increasing, but it was waiting to be sealed and to become fame; and, as she says herself, it was the greatest French poet of the century who was to crown her with the laurel of the elect.

This happened in 1872, when Victor Hugo's *Ruy Blas* was revived at the Odéon. The first night was on 26th January.

She rehearsed the play with Victor Hugo himself. She played the part of the Queen: Maria de Neubourg. It was her first great poetic creation. By her own account she must have been trying at rehearsal, surrounded as she was at that time by flatterers, and she went out of her way to irritate the poet; but she tells us that he defeated her by his good nature, and that, after the first performance was over, there was nothing but complete satisfaction between the poet who had seen his dream incarnate and the actress who knew she had done well.

Writing of her performance in this part when the play was produced at the Odéon, Sarcey said that Mademoiselle Sarah Bernhardt had received from nature the gift of wearied and melancholy dignity. Every motion she made was noble and harmonious; whether she got up or sat down, whether she walked or half turned, the long folds of her gown laced with silver hung around her with a poetical grace. 'The voice is languishing and tender, her delivery so true in rhythm and so clear in utterance that never a syllable is lost, even when the words float from her lips like a caress. And how marvellously she follows the curve of a speech, letting it unfurl without a break, maintaining the harmony of its flexible line. And with what delicate and telling intonation she underlines certain words, giving them an extraordinary value.'[1]

Later on, when the same play was done at the Théâtre Français in 1879, Sarcey spoke again of her charm, her languorous grace and tenderness in this part; of the delicate demure fun with which she spoke certain lines, of the passion which she suggested. 'But all that,' he said, 'is still not the best part of her success. In what does it reside? Well, her triumph was that she sang, yes, chanted with her melodious voice those verses which are wafted like the sighs that the wind draws from an Aeolian harp:

> Blessé! Qui que tu sois, ô jeune homme inconnu,
> Toi, qui me voyant seule, et loin de ce que j'aime,
> Sans me rien demander, sans rien espérer même,

[1] Sarcey, *La Comédie Française*.

SARAH BERNHARDT

Viens à moi, sans compter les périls où tu cours;
Toi qui verses ton sang et qui risques tes jours
Pour donner une fleur à la reine d'Espagne;
Qui que tu sois, ami dont l'ombre m'accompagne,
Puisque mon cœur subit une inflexible loi,
Sois aimé par ta mère et sois béni par moi!

'This lovely lullaby was sighed in melting accents by Mademoiselle Sarah Bernhardt; she did not attempt any effects of light or shade; it was a long caress of sound which had in its very monotony something dulcet and penetrating; all she did was to add the music of her voice to the music of the verse.'[1]

This is how Théodore de Banville described her appearance at that moment:

'She is the only player whom the Creator had fashioned solely for the art of play-acting: tall as Rosalind, slender enough for any disguise, she is in so high a degree poetry incarnate that even when she is still and mute we are aware that her gait as well as her voice is subservient to a lyrical rhythm. A Greek sculptor seeking a symbol for the Ode would have chosen her for a model. A great actress should be able to play Juliet and Lady Macbeth, Iphigénie and Ériphile, Chimène and Pauline; consequently

[1] Sarcey, *Quarante Ans de Théâtre*, vol. iv, p. 54.

SARAH BERNHARDT

she must be neither dark nor fair. Thus Sarah Bernhardt, with her beautiful Dutch colouring, is neither fair nor dark. If she sprinkles her hair with water, it is fair; pomade turns it brown, and it is so naturally curled and waved and so fuzzy and frizzled, in so wondrous a shock, in so Goddess-like a mane, like the tresses of Diane de Poitiers intermingled by the sculptor Jean Goujon, that she has only to ruffle it and plunge a pin into it to change it into the most elegant and complex of head-dresses. Heinrich Heine should have known her when he sang Hérodiade in his *Atta Troll,* how devoutly he would have used that face as a model! the face of a Queen of Cappadocia, or of a Nereid, evoking the pearly shell of the ocean: the narrow forehead, with its very soft and very bright skin, the eyebrows rather close together and thickening towards the nose, long, deeply-carved brown eyes, half-closed, and as a rule listless, but when she comes to life awakening and glinting like black diamonds; the pupil so very small, and yet when the actress lets fly a shaft of irony it seems to leap from the eyes and to pierce you; the nose is semitic, but turned to grace by a curve of the nostril, as if uplifted by the little ridge in its midst, that signifies poetry and the fighting spirit: nor must we forget the clear-cut resolute chin, the gracious mouth with its incarnadined and delicate lips opening on a dazzling and fierce array of white teeth; and to the end of time the image of Sarah Bernhardt will be evoked whenever Ruy Blas shall say

> 'She wore a little crown of silver lace.'
>
> ('Elle avait un petit diadème en dentelle d'argent.')

She was described at this epoch of her career as being impalpable—*c'était une fumée, une vapeur* (Felicia Mallet), and Matthew Arnold sums it all up when he talks of a fugitive vision of delicate features under a shower of hair and a cloud of lace. She was so thin that people laughed at her, and one of the jokes of the time was that an empty carriage drew up at the door, 'and out jumped Sarah Bernhardt.'[1]

It was after her performance in *Ruy Blas* and her triumph in the part of the Queen that she was offered an engagement at the Théâtre Fran-

---

[1] 'How wonderful she looked in those days! She was as transparent as an azalea, only more so; like a cloud, only not so thick. Smoke from a burning paper describes her more nearly! She was hollow-eyed, thin, almost consumptive-looking. Her body was not the prison of her soul, but its shadow.'—Ellen Terry, *Memoirs*.

çais, and signed it without consulting the manager of the Odéon, where she was playing. He brought an action against her, and she had to pay 6000 francs damages: the first of several experiences of this kind. She left the Odéon, with regret, and made her début at the Français in a play of Alexandre Dumas *père*, *Mademoiselle de Belle-Isle*. This first night was on 6th November 1872. She suffered, as she always did throughout her life on first nights, from stage fright; and she was not a success, save towards the end. Only in two passages, Sarcey said, was the Sarah of *Ruy Blas* recognisable. 'I doubt,' he said, 'whether Mademoiselle Sarah Bernhardt will ever be able, with her delicious voice, to render those deep, thrilling notes, and to express the paroxysms of violent passion that carry an audience away. If nature had endowed her with that gift she would be a perfect artist, and such a thing does not exist on the stage.'[1]

After that she appeared as Junie in Racine's *Britannicus*, in which part Sarcey said she had '*je ne sais quel charme poétique, elle dit le vers avec une grâce et une pureté Raciniennes*'; as Chérubin in *Le Mariage de Figaro* in 1873

[1] Sarcey, *Le Temps*, 11th November 1872.

(30th January); in Octave Feuillet's *Dalila* on 28th March 1873; and in *Andromaque* in August 1873. Then, in September 1873, she played the small part of Aricie in *Phèdre*. But already seeds of friction were beginning to grow. There was jealousy between her and the leading comedy actress, Croizette, who was given the best parts. She was entitled to the leading parts in comedy, as she was, according to all accounts, a first-rate interpreter of what the French call high comedy; but Sarah was burning for her chance, for an opportunity of showing what she could do, and she did not care whether this were to be in tragedy or comedy, for she was ready to do both. Sarah wanted to play in Musset's *On ne badine pas avec l'amour*. She wanted to play Célimène. The parts were given to Croizette, and rightly. The management refused to yield these parts to Sarah, who on her side began to lose interest, or to feign to lose interest, in her work, and took to sculpture. The management became alarmed, and gave her a part to create in a new play by Octave Feuillet. The principal part was given to Croizette, but Sarah was pleased with her secondary part, and determined it should be equally important, if not more important than the principal part. And here it may be said that from the very beginning to the very end of her career nobody was ever more absolutely certain of what she could do and what she could not do, and whether or no she could make something or nothing of a part; and those who persuaded her to act against her instinct in these matters invariably lived to regret it.

After stormy rehearsals, this play, *Le Sphinx*, was a success (23rd March 1874); as Sarah had foreseen, although Croizette was triumphant, her own success was the more keenly appreciated by the critical. Sarah then asked for a holiday; it was refused. She was to play in Voltaire's *Zaïre*. The first night was to be on 6th August 1874. It was a tropically hot summer; rehearsals lasted throughout June and July. Sarah, who did not wish to play, swore that since they wished it, she would play, but die. She played in the stifling heat; and she had made up her mind to faint, to bleed, and to die in earnest, to spite Perrin, the director of the Français. She played with every fibre of her body. She sobbed and suffered in earnest. When she was stabbed on the stage she uttered a real cry of suffering, as she thought she was dying. To her immense astonishment, when the curtain fell she found she was able to take her call with ease, and felt strong enough to begin the whole performance over again. This was a critical turning-point in her career, perhaps the most critical of all. She knew now that she could draw when she liked and as she liked upon her physical resources; and she realised, too, another thing. Hitherto she had been acclaimed as a charming, frail and poetic vision. She was thought to have a delicate constitution and weak lungs; she did not expect to live long; and it was taken for granted that she was without strength or authority, either as a woman or an artist; and now, from this moment, knowing that she could count on the strength of her vocal cords, and that her supply of electric energy was inexhaustible, she resolved to be strong, and to live to the utmost and to the end, and she put away from her all thoughts of an early death.

This performance revealed to her her own incredible energy. She could rehearse all day, and play an arduous part at night; or play all day and rehearse all night. She never needed a rest, and, while strong men in her company crumbled and succumbed around her, and threw up the sponge, she remained at her post, fresh as a daisy; and this was the manner of her routine until she died in 1923 at the age of 79.

After some months of inaction, the death of a sister, an illness, and a journey to Nice with her son (for now she had a son), Perrin offered her the part of Phèdre, which on the French stage is the most arduous and difficult, the most important of all parts, and is to a French actress what the part of Hamlet is to an English actor. The performance took place on the anniversary of Racine's birthday, 21st December 1874. She accepted the part with trepidation. She studied it with Regnier, once a famous actor, whose pupil she had been, and who had been a professor at the Conservatoire. He told her there was nothing for her to be afraid of; all she had to do was to be careful not to force her voice, and to play the part in sorrow rather than in frenzy, which would be no loss to anybody—not even to Racine.

On the first night she was half-dead with stage fright, but she regained her self-control just before going on; the performance was a triumph for her, and she was almost unanimously praised by the Press. Those who saw her and Rachel in this part said that Sarah was equal, if not superior to Rachel in the first three acts, but inferior to her in the last two. Of the first night Sarcey wrote:

'She compelled the old connoisseurs to admit that in the second act at least she was equal to the memories of the great tragédienne. *Phèdre* set the seal on her reputation, which from now onwards is fame. It is true that she will never play the fourth act with the energy and pace that the interpretation of these high passions demands; but in the first three acts she is incomparable, and I have heard many good judges admit that in these she is more completely satisfying than her great predecessor.' [1]

Twenty years later Sarcey changed his mind about her playing in the last two acts. He thought her then exceedingly fine in these as well. Perhaps the explanation is merely that she was older. For, according to all accounts, although her playing of this part, her 'conception' of it, never really varied, it nevertheless gained in authority: and, when she played it

[1] *La Comédie Française.*

twenty or twenty-five years later, there was a power and strength in the last two acts which only age and experience could give. The plastic and musical beauty of the creation was the same as it had always been.

Soon after this she created a part in a poetic play called *La Fille de Roland* (15th February 1875), in which, contrary to expectation, she triumphed; and then Alexandre Dumas *fils* announced to her one day that he had a part ready for her in a new modern play which he was to produce at the Théâtre Français, called *L'Étrangère*. Sarah was told she was to play the part of the Duchess, which seemed to be the chief part; but when the parts were distributed she received that of Mistress Clarkson, who was L'Étrangère. Sarah was delighted, for she preferred this so-called secondary part, and she resolved, and managed, to make it the more important of the two; and, after some stormy rehearsals, the play was produced (14th February 1876) with great success, of which she was the centre, turning the rather tawdry melodrama of her part into bright gold.

That same year she exhibited a group of sculpture in the Salon, and about a month later, after the opening of this exhibition, there was a reading at the Comédie Française of a drama in verse called *Rome Vaincue* by Parodi. Sarah was offered the part of the heroine, a Vestal, Opimia, but she refused it and chose instead the part of an old blind woman, the Vestal's grandmother, who, to save her grand-daughter, guilty of breaking her vow, from being buried alive, has to kill her. The Vestal is bound and cannot stab herself, and the blind grandmother has to fumble for the place of her heart. This was one of the most striking instances of how right Sarah was to follow her own instinct. For the first time she revealed to the public something of the wide range of her electric power and dramatic imagination.

The play was produced on 27th September 1876. Sarcey, in writing about her, says that 'she revealed qualities of energy and pathos which even her warmest admirers did not suspect; she was admirably dressed and made up; a drawn, wrinkled face of extraordinary majesty; vague and lifeless eyes; a cloak which fell on both sides, and when she lifted her arms seemed like the immense wings of some enormous and sinister bat. Nothing could be more terrible or at the same time more poetical. It was no longer an actress who was there; it was Nature herself, with a marvellous understanding at her service, a soul of fire, and the truest and most melodious voice that has ever charmed mortal ear. This woman plays with her heart and her inmost being; she dares gestures that would be ridiculous in another, and which bring down the house.' [1]

Years afterwards she played an act of this play at her jubilee performance at the Renaissance, and I have been told by several of her greatest admirers that never in her whole career did she produce so profound an effect as when the blind grandmother groped and fumbled for the Vestal's heart so as to stab her.

Her next great success, which was another definite landmark in her career, was the revival of Victor Hugo's *Hernani* on 21st November 1877. Once more she rehearsed a play with Victor Hugo himself. Mounet-Sully played Hernani, and Worms Charles v. She was destined to more startling successes in her career, but probably never revealed to the public a more delicate incarnation than her rendering

[1] *Quarante Ans de Théâtre.*

of Doña Sol. This sealed her success at the Théâtre Français, which was blazing all through the period of the Paris Exhibition in 1878.

Victor Hugo, writing to her after the first night, said: *'Vous avez été grande et charmante; vous m'avez ému, moi le vieux combatteur, et à un certain moment, pendant que le public attendri et enchanté par vous applaudissait, j'ai pleuré. Cette larme que vous avez fait couler est à vous.'*

She was now famous: throughout this time her relations with the management of the Théâtre Français were becoming more and more strained. Her successes caused exasperation as well as pleasure in some quarters; and her fits of wilfulness, her whims, her hobbies, her sculpture, her flight in a balloon (surely harmless enough), the publicity which began to gather round her name, irritated the director of the classic theatre. In April 1879 she reappeared in her part as the Queen in *Ruy Blas*, and that summer the whole of the Comédie Française paid a visit to London.

Sarah Bernhardt had in one sense reached the zenith of her career. In the interpretation of poetry, classic or romantic, she had reached the high-water mark of her art. She never did anything better in poetic art than Phèdre, Andromaque, Doña Sol, and the Queen in *Ruy Blas*. But, in spite of this, she had not yet begun to show all she could do. She had not struck all the chords of her lyre. Nor had her personality and her genius matured to the full. She was destined to greater efforts, wider conquests, and more sensational effects; she was to strike harder and more deeply, but she was never to be more perfect or more poetical: never so perfect, some say. She was acting good plays the whole time; she was always interpreting good literature, and sometimes divine poetry. She was putting life into Racine, she was rendering Victor Hugo's verse as it has never been interpreted before or since; Doña Sol was perhaps the part in which she attained the highest poetical perfection. Phèdre was more wonderful, but there were moments in her Phèdre at that date, so it seems, when the mantle of the part was too heavy for her delicate frame and mechanism; and when she acted the part years later, in the full maturity of her genius, there were moments when her voice showed signs of strain and rust; but in the seventies and eighties, in Victor Hugo's

SARAH BERNHARDT

Hernani and *Ruy Blas,* she had poetry, passion, and grace and youth, and first love to express. She expressed it easily, with unerring poetical tact; there was no strain, not a harsh note, it was a symphony of golden flutes and muted strings; a summer dawn lit by lambent lightnings, soft stars, and a clear-cut crescent moon.

CHAPTER III

SARAH BERNHARDT came to London with the whole company of the Comédie Francaise. It was a marvellous cast, and they brought with them a fine repertory of plays, ancient and modern. The cast consisted of Got, the Coquelin brothers, Worms, Croizette, Baretta, Fèbre, etc. They gave forty-three performances, and plays by Molière, Racine, Beaumarchais, Victor Hugo, Alexandre Dumas *fils,* Georges Sand, Feuillet, Augier, Musset, Sandeau, Coppée, Balzac, etc., and Sarah Bernhardt played in eighteen of these. She played in *Phèdre, L'Étrangère, Le Sphinx, Hernani;* her performances gave an average of 13,350 francs each, while the twenty-five other performances gave an average of 10,000 francs each. Besides this, she acted in scenes and short plays in private houses.

She became instantly the fashion and the rage. More than the rage, the shibboleth of the intellectuals, and the catchword of the world of fashion. Years later, in 1896, Eleonora Duse, during her second season in London (during the first, in 1893, she had played to empty houses), became the shibboleth of the London intelligentsia, and they compared her with Sarah Bernhardt, to the disadvantage of the latter; but they seemed unaware that they were comparing the summer tide of one artist with the autumn of the other, and they had forgotten or knew not that London had gone madder over Sarah Bernhardt's spring than ever they had over Duse's summer.

Sarah's success in London was universal. It was not only startling; it was comprehensive. London went mad over the whole French players in general, but especially mad over Sarah. Matthew Arnold writes an interesting article about it:

'From time to time,' he says, 'France or things French become for the solid English public the object of what our neighbours call an *enjouement* [sic]—an infatuated interest. . . .

> Lords, lawyers, statesmen, squires of low degree,
> Men known and men unknown.

The rush of those acquainted with the French language perfectly, of those acquainted with it little, and of those not acquainted with it at all, to the performances at the Gaiety Theatre, the length and solemnity with which the newspapers chronicled and discussed them, the seriousness with which the whole repertory was taken, the passion for certain pieces and for certain actors, the great ladies who by the acting of Mademoiselle Sarah Bernhardt were revealed to themselves, and who could not resist the desire of telling her so, all this has moved, I say, a surviving and aged moralist here and there amongst us to exclaim:

Shame on you, feeble heads, to slavery prone! . . .'

The centre of this rage was without doubt Sarah Bernhardt. She was the lioness of the moment, eclipsing all others on the stage and off. The following episode illustrated by du Maurier appeared in *Punch*. The picture represented a club, and two elegant young men talking to each other, and an old fogey looking at them from the distance with surprised disgust. Underneath the picture, which is called 'The Divine Sarah,' is the following dialogue:

First Critic (aetat. 21): 'Beats Rachel hollow in Ong-dromack, hanged if she don't!'

Second Critic (ditto): 'So I think, old man! And in L'Etronjair she licks Mademoiselle Mars all to fits!'

Punch was full of her doings. Here is the first stanza of a typical poem, published in its columns at this moment:

> Mistress of Hearts and Arts, all met in you!
>   The picturesque, informed by soul of Passion!
> Say, dost thou feed on milk and honey-dew,
>   Draining from goblets deep of classic fashion
> Champagne and nectar, shandy-gaff sublime,
>   Dashed with a pungent smack of Eau-de-Marah,
> Aspasia, Sappho, Circe of the time!
>   Seductive Sarah!

The vogue included the great public as well as the élite of the intellectuals, and the world of society and fashion. London went simply mad, but Sarah had to pay a price for this infatuation. The public was not so fastidious as the French. Matthew Arnold by his criticisms of French verse in his article proved he did not understand French, and he even got the word for infatuation, which he chooses to quote in French, wrong, calling it *enjouement*, which means 'liveliness.'

Sarah insisted in making her first appearance

SARAH BERNHARDT

in London in the second act of *Phèdre,* and, as always happened when confronted with a friendly audience, she was panic-stricken by stage fright, and had to be pushed on to the stage.

She was nervous on that occasion, and on first nights the occasion often repeated itself: nearly always, she once told me, when she knew the audience was friendly; but never in later life, when she expected the audience to be hostile; then to the end of her life, when she felt herself about to confront all that was most critical in Paris, to set a dish before palates that were jaded, and admirers who had long ago tired of her, and critics who were definitely hostile—then every fibre in her being was tautened for the fight, and all shadow of nervousness left her. On the other hand, when the audience was friendly, she felt deprived of her power, weak and helpless, and without that asset Henry James so beautifully defines in *The Tragic Muse:* 'the perfect presence of mind, unconfused, unhurried by emotion, that any artistic performance requires, and that all, whatever the instrument, require exactly in the same degree: the application, in other words, clear, and calculated, crystal-firm, as it were, of the idea conceived in the glow of experience.'

I would add, in Sarah Bernhardt's case, unconsciously conceived.

Ellen Terry says somewhere: 'The actor must imagine first and observe afterwards. It is no good observing life and then bringing the result to the stage without selection, without a definite idea. The idea must come first, the realism afterwards.' This, I believe, describes what Sarah Bernhardt did; she imagined first, that is to say she guessed by instinct; if she had 'conceptions' of her parts, she formed these afterwards, *après coup*. But she never spoke of conceptions of a part in private, and in public only in print, that is to say in self-defence, when her reading of a part was challenged or attacked.

To go back to the first night of *Phèdre*. This is how she tells the story:

'The time came for me to go on. I had the *trac* (stage-fright), not the kind that paralyses but the kind that makes one lose one's head. That is bad enough, but preferable; one does too much, but one does something. The whole house had clapped my entry for several minutes; and as I bent down in recognition of the homage I said to myself, "Yes, yes, you will see. I will give you my blood—my life . . . my soul." And as I started my scene, I was not entirely in possession of myself, I took the speech a shade too high. It was impossible to lower the pitch once I had begun. I was off, nothing could stop me. I suffered. I wept. I beseeched. I cried out; and all was genuine. My suffering was atrocious; I shed burning and bitter tears. I besought Hippolyte for the love that was slaying me, and the arms which I stretched out to Mounet-Sully were the arms of Phèdre contorted by cruel desire. The god was there. When the curtain fell Mounet-Sully carried me away senseless to my dressing-room.'[1]

The English Press was lyrical. The following extract from the *Standard* is typical. 'The subdued passion, repressed for a time until at length it burst its bonds, and a despairing heart-broken woman is revealed to Hippolyte, was shown with so vivid a reality that a scene of enthusiasm such as is rarely witnessed in the theatre followed the fall of the curtain.'

[1] *Ma Double Vie*, vol. ii, p. 106.

SARAH BERNHARDT

The *Morning Post* said: 'As her passion mastered what remained of modesty and reserve in her nature, the woman sprang forward and recoiled again with the movement of a panther, striving as it seemed to tear from her bosom the heart which stifled her with its unholy longing, until in the end, when terrified at the horror her breathings have provoked in Hippolyte, she strove to pull his sword from its sheath and plunge it in her own breast, she fell in complete and absolute collapse. This exhibition, marvellous in beauty of pose, in febrile force, in intensity, in purity of delivery, is the more remarkable as the passion had to be reached, so to speak, at a bound, no performance of the first act having raised the actress to the requisite heat.'

But this is how Sarcey tells the story:

'She took, as is natural in moments of great emotion, her first note too high, and once having started on that pitch, as experienced actors know well, she had to keep it up. She had to start from the high note and rise higher as the sentiment she had to express became stronger and more pathetic. She was obliged to scream. She hurried her delivery. She was lost. You think perhaps the English audience experienced that sense of discomfort we should have felt in Paris? On the contrary they were delighted, applauding with frenzy, and when she re-appeared half dead on the arm of Mounet-Sully they made her an ovation. The next evening, not yet recovered, and out of temper with herself and everyone else, she appeared as Mrs. Clarkson in *L'Étrangère* and only gave a relative idea of what she could do with that part. She might have saved herself any trouble. She could have splashed about in the part as she pleased. The audience had made up its mind to admire her, and this enthusiasm was reflected in the Press. . . . What will they say when they really see her act well, for she can act very well?'

Not one of the English critics noticed what had happened to her on that first night, and a few days later she left out a whole speech, one of the most important speeches, in the part of Mrs. Clarkson, without a soul noticing it. Henceforth Sarah must have known that her task when faced by a foreign audience was easier than when she was faced by the pitilessly observant and mercilessly critical Parisians, whom not a shade or inflection or intonation, nor any false note or lifting of an eyelash, escaped. The door was opened for her now, not only on triumph, but on easy triumph; and easy triumph cannot help being detrimental to art. It is remarkable that Sarah's art came as scatheless as it did through so many easy triumphs, and the reason is perhaps that it was yearly, or once every two years, checked by a dose of Paris; and her greatest triumphs of all were those which she won before a Parisian audience; especially before a Parisian audience that had made up its mind to be hostile. There is not an instance in her whole career when she did not defeat such hostility.

The astounding vogue she enjoyed in London inevitably marshalled all the demons and jackals of publicity. Sarah was advertised, paragraphed, caricatured, gossiped about. Innumerable legends grew up about her. It was said she had tamed lions. That she had broken a boxing instructor's teeth, and that she dressed up as a man (she did wear a pair of white trousers when doing sculpture). The Parisian newspapers repeated these rumours with scathing comment, dictated sometimes by envy.

Caricature was busy. Her extreme thinness was still a constant topic of the paragraphists and subject of caricature. She was drawn as a stick with a sponge at the top of it. The *Figaro* attacked her for her eccentricities, and Sarah answered by telegram, saying that if the stories told about her annoyed the public, and they had decided to receive her ungraciously, she would send in her resignation, as she did not wish anyone to act so basely on her account. Her colleagues begged her to reconsider her decision, and Sarah listened to them. She returned to Paris. She was well received the first time she appeared at the Français, and all seemed well; but all was not well. She was given a part in a new play by Emile Augier, *L'Aventurière*—a play in verse. Augier was an excellent playwright, but he was not only not a poet, he had not a spark of poetry in his composition. Sarah, whose instincts as an actress were highly responsive to verse, felt this instantly. She detested the play, despised the verse, and hated her part.

The play was performed on 17th April 1880. Sarah had just recovered from a cold, her dress did not suit her, she was still rather hoarse.

She played feebly and looked ill. She was in a bad temper. The Press attacked her, and accused her of vulgarity of gesture. She shut herself up all the morning, and then, after much deliberation, she sent in her resignation from the Comédie Française to the Director, Monsieur Perrin, and sent copies of it to the Press, lest it be refused. She left Paris and went to Havre. The Comédie Française brought an action against her claiming 300,000 francs damages, and the loss of 43,000 francs, which she was owed. She lost her suit and had to find these sums.

Three days after her resignation an American, Jarrett, called on her and proposed to take her to America on an extensive tour. He had made this proposal to her two or three times before, but she had refused it. The terms he proposed were as follows: 5000 francs for each performance, and half of the receipts above 15,000 francs; *i.e.* 7500 francs if the receipts reached 20,000 francs. In addition, 1000 a week for her hotel bills, a special Pullman car on all railway journeys, with bedroom and drawing-room for herself and her staff, and two cooks. Mr. Jarrett was to get 10 per cent. of all sums. She accepted at once. Jarrett at once cabled to Mr. Abbey, the American impresario, who agreed. Thirteen days later the contract was signed: she was given 10,000 francs in advance, she was to play seven plays—*Hernani, Phèdre, Adrienne Lecouvreur, Froufrou, La Dame aux Camélias, L'Étrangère, La Princesse Georges.*

Such is the story of the obvious and palpable reasons which caused Sarah Bernhardt to leave the Français and to become a world star.

This crossing of the ways, which cut her whole career in two, and which took place in Paris, was probably, consciously or unconsciously, caused by what happened in London. Sarah, after her return to Paris and her want of success in *L'Aventurière,* had to choose between a comparatively quiet life of repertory at the Théâtre Français, and an adventurous life of individual effort all over the world; and as is usual in such crises, where choice is inevitable, there were probably two motives at work: the superficial, obvious motive, which seems to be imperatively guiding the person along one course, and towards one goal, and the hidden motive, which sometimes, unknown to the chooser himself, is in reality the guide and guardian, and the determining factor. In this case, and at this moment, the superficial motives were the friction and breach between Sarah and her colleagues of the Comédie Française, and her quarrel with the Director; and this friction was increased, if not brought about, by Sarah's astounding vogue in London in 1879; but probably, unseen by the world and only dimly guessed at by herself, there were deeper reasons, the reasons of nature and Providence; an unbridled love of adventure, an insatiable curiosity, a thirst of conquest and a desire of new worlds to conquer. But deeper than all this and stronger than all this, was the need of self-expression, of giving to the full and to the utmost the whole gamut of music which she knew was concealed in the frail yet steel-like instrument of her being. For the season in London had taught her that she had as yet expressed only a small part of what she divined she was able to do.

CHAPTER IV

To the end of her career there were critics who deplored her leaving the Théâtre Français, and who were never tired of beseeching her to go back to it. The truth is, she was working out her own salvation in the only way in which it was possible for her to do so. She was following her instincts, and she was right. In the article which I have already quoted, Matthew Arnold writes about her as follows:

'One remark I will make, a remark suggested by the inevitable comparison of Mademoiselle Sarah Bernhardt with Rachel—one talks vaguely of genius, but I have never till now comprehended how much of Rachel's superiority was purely intellectual power, how eminently this power counts in the actor's art, as in all art; how just is the instinct which led the Greeks to mark with a high and severe stamp the Muses. Temperament and quick intelligence, passion, nervous mobility, grace, smile, voice, charm, poetry—Mademoiselle Sarah Bernhardt has them all. One watches her with pleasure, with admiration—and yet not without a secret disquietude. Something is wanting, or at least not present in sufficient force; something which alone can secure and fix her administration of all the charming gifts which she has, can alone keep them fresh, keep them sincere, save them from perils by caprice, perils by mannerism. That something is high intellectual power. It was here that Rachel was so great; she began, one says to oneself, as one recalls her majesty and dwells upon it—she began almost where Mademoiselle Sarah Bernhardt ends.'

I believe that when Matthew Arnold wrote this criticism it was a just one, although the phrase 'intellectual power' is really a misnomer: the wrong phrase for the right idea. It is on record that Rachel was totally unacquainted with some of the finest portions of a play of Corneille's in which she acted.[1] She had never bothered to read a whole act in which she did not appear. She did not know how the play ended. This, if true, was not of the slightest consequence. I do not believe that Rachel, or

[1] 'Nous ne voudrions en rien diminuer sa gloire, mais là était l'originalité de son talent; Mademoiselle Rachel fut plutôt une mime tragique qu'une tragédienne.'—Théophile Gautier, 1858.

Sarah, or Duse, or Salvini, or Irving, or indeed any actor, had a shred of intellectual power; but they had the power of genius and the instinct of doing the right thing in the right way, so that you had the illusion that this was due to intellectual power. And when Matthew Arnold says that Rachel began almost where Sarah Bernhardt ended, I believe he was again right at this moment; but it might be said that it turned out later that Sarah's real greatness began where the Sarah of the seventies ended.

Before she left America she proved that she could show to the public facets of her genius for which the Théâtre Français had hitherto given her no scope, and which were yet undreamt of by the public and by the critics. Before leaving for America she gave a season in London, where she acted all the plays she was to play in America. The French critics came to London to see these performances. They were already angry with her, and were prepared to be angrier. 'We have heard enough of Mademoiselle Sarah Bernhardt,' Vitu wrote in the *Figaro*. 'Let her go abroad with her monotonous voice and her morbid whims; we have nothing new to learn from her talents or her caprices.'

'Morbid whims' was an allusion to her having had herself photographed in a coffin during the time when she felt she was due for an early death.

Sarcey, writing of her resignation from the Français, ended up by saying:

'There comes a time when naughty children must be sent to bed.'

The critics came to curse: but they stayed to bless.

She opened her season with *Adrienne Lecouvreur*. Auguste Vitu's report was as follows:

'The sincerity of my admiration cannot be doubted when I confess that in the fifth act Sarah Bernhardt rose to a height of dramatic power, to a force of expression, which could not be surpassed. She played the long and cruel scene in which the poisoned Adrienne struggles against death in her fearful agony, not only with immense talent, but with an artistic science which up to the present she has never revealed.'

Sarcey was still more dithyrambic; in his article in the *Temps* of 31st May 1880, he reports that the public were slightly cold at first, but were taken captive as soon as Sarah spoke the lines of La Fontaine's fable; and although in the following act she missed some of the stock points in the play, in the last act she swept the audience and the critics off their feet. It is the scene where she lies poisoned by the flowers sent her by her rival. 'It was a combination,' he wrote, 'of the most harrowing truth and the most delicate idealism. She would have drawn tears in this scene from a stone; and one felt a certain pleasure in shedding these tears, as happens whenever human sorrows, instead of finding crude expression, as they do in real life, come to us softened by the cunning medium of art.

'There were no screams, no contortions, no grimaces. Everything was poignant, chaste, noble and harmonious. I do not fancy that it has ever been our lot to witness anything more perfect; never has truth been seen to soar higher on the wings of poetry.

'The English audience applauded loudly; not enough, in my opinion. Ah, if Mademoiselle Sarah Bernhardt had played that fifth act at Paris, what enthusism there would have been! What raptures! And the next day what a torrent of praise in the newspapers!'

This performance, and these criticisms, show

not only that Sarah had revealed something she had never shown before, but she had done something for which the Théâtre Français would have given her no scope. The performance was followed by that of *Froufrou,* in which she had to compete with the memories, still fresh, of Aimée Desclée, an actress of genius who had played the part in London not many years before. This was a formidable handicap, because Desclée, who had since died in her prime, had identified herself with the part of the wayward child of Paris, so foolish, so frivolous, so fond and so irresistible, with the grace of a kitten and the frailty of porcelain, the butterfly broken on a cruel wheel. Théodore de Banville wrote about Desclée thus:

'Above all things she is more of a woman than all other women put together; panting and hungry-eyed, she herself challenges the serpent beneath the tree and beseeches him in broken accents full of anguish: "Won't you tell me where I can find the apple?" And no sooner has she eaten of the apple than in sobs and tears she convinces Adam that it is his fault. . . . Burn the whole of the *Comédie Humaine,* obliterate all we know of modern life, let oblivion swallow all the long stories of all forsaken maidens, the martyrdoms of wives, the loves of great ladies who love like the Gods in a region forbidden and aloof from ordinary mortals . . . cancel the betrayals, the passions, the frenzy, the patient resignation, the desperate aspirations, the hate, the fury, the delirious ecstasy, and you will find the whole epoch in the staring pupils and trembling lips of Aimée Desclée.'

There are playgoers still alive who have told me that they saw Aimée Desclée play that part, and that they could not imagine anyone comparing Sarah Bernhardt with her. Such, however, was not the opinion of Francisque Sarcey, who wrote of Sarah's performance when that of Desclée was still in his memory: so fresh that he could compare the performances detail by detail. I will quote his opinion presently.

Froufrou is a light comedy ending in tragedy. It was the *Doll's House* of its day, though of the two plays perhaps that of Ibsen seems the more old-fashioned. This is the fate of all plays that startle more by the modernity of their ideas than by their truth to nature. It is a brilliant picture of contemporary manners and drama, of Parisian life in the sixties. The play can still be read with pleasure, and could be acted with success were there an actress anywhere who could play the part. It is the story of a light woman, light as gossamer, a child of Paris and of candlelight: a child of the Second Empire; frivolous, gay, harmless, anxious to give and to receive pleasure, and above all things pretty. She has a seriously-minded sister, and she marries a seriously-minded husband, with the possibilities of a career, who adores her. The sister comes to live with them after their marriage (the sister had loved the husband before Froufrou was married, but had said nothing about it, and the husband is unaware of this fact). Gradually and fatally, what with Froufrou's many engagements, her invitations, her presence at balls, parties, exhibitions, suppers, plays, and private theatricals, the daily affairs of the family, and the care of her child, devolve on her sister Louise, who, conscientiously and without a shadow of bad faith, fulfils all the duties that Froufrou leaves undone, and sees to all the practical side of the household and the nursery. One fine day Froufrou realises too late that it is Louise who is performing the part of wife and mother in the house, and not she at all. At once she becomes a prey to jealousy, and there is a scene in the third act when the sisters quarrel, or rather when Froufrou forces a quarrel on her patient sister and accuses her of treachery and of having robbed her of her husband. Froufrou in a rage finally explodes at the end of a long, slow, and gradual crescendo of recrimination. And anyone who has ever taken part in a real quarrel, or witnessed one in real life, when they saw Sarah's performance of that scene must have been staggered by the supreme beauty, the subtle truth, and inspired realism in the rendering of that moment when the little rift is seen gradually to widen, almost before you are aware, into an unbridgeable gulf, and to end in irretrievable disaster.

When I saw Sarah play the scene of this quarrel (many years later, in the nineties), it was like watching someone skating on thin ice and knowing that they are getting nearer and nearer to peril; like watching a glass being filled drop by drop and knowing that the moment will come when the water will overflow. It was the overtones of her play here that were so wonderful. The slight indication she gave of what was going on, and of all that had been going on beneath the surface for months; a slow and gradually rippling tide of irritation indicated now by a tremble in the finger, a certain recklessness, a catch in the voice, or a twitch of the shoulder, and an ominous glinting of the eyes, merging fast into exasperation, that was now about to explode, and did explode in an outburst of vituperation, jealousy, and unbridled blinding passion. The effect on the audience was all the more remarkable from the gradual way in which the explosion was led up to.

Sarcey does not say that Sarah was superior to Desclée. After describing Desclée playing the scene in the third act, when Froufrou attacks her sister, saying that she strode up and down the stage with long strides, shaking her head like a furious and runaway colt, hurling in broken phrases the bitterest reproaches at her sister, while her sister ran after her pulling at her gown, and unable to say anything except 'Gilberte! Gilberte!' 'How' (Sarcey asks himself) 'could Mademoiselle Sarah Bernhardt act such a scene, she whose movements are disciplined, she who is a living harmony, a lyric in flesh and blood?

'Well! She succeeded. It is a different thing,

but it is just as powerful. Mademoiselle Sarah Bernhardt stands upright, almost immobile, down stage, facing the public, when she hurls the terrible accusation: "Ah! How well you knew how to make me will what you willed! How clever you are, sister! What a child I am compared with you!" etc. But the movement which the other actress expressed in her arms and in her legs, how thoroughly Mademoiselle Sarah Bernhardt conveyed it in her voice. What extraordinary fullness she gave to her grievances and her recriminations.[1]

'I do not wish to say that Mademoiselle Sarah Bernhardt has obliterated the memory of Mademoiselle Desclée, because it is impossible to choose between two interpretations so absolutely different and equally perfect, nor can we give the palm to one or the other.

'The manner of stirring the audience has changed, but the emotion is the same in kind: deep, amazing, incredible. The applause was frantic, and the actress was recalled three times.

[1] It is interesting to notice that her playing of the scene as described by Sarcey in 1880 is different from that which I describe, and which I saw many years later. By that time Sarah was considerably older, confessedly too old for the first act, and was husbanding her means, and played almost the whole scene sitting down.

'... In the fourth act there is no possible discussion. Mademoiselle Sarah Bernhardt showed herself superior to her predecessor. In this act drama, or if you prefer it high tragedy, breaks in. Nothing for those who were not present at this astonishing performance can give any idea of the heart-rending cries of Froufrou as she throws her arms round her husband's neck to prevent him going to fight a duel,—I don't think that in the theatre emotion has ever reached so poignant a pitch. There are in the art of the stage these exceptional moments when artists are transported out of themselves, beyond themselves, and do better than their best, in obedience to the dictates of some familiar spirit or *daimon* such as Corneille used to say whispered rhymes into his ears.'[1]

The last sentence of this criticism is particularly interesting because Sarah herself used to say, and I have heard her say it often, after a performance she was satisfied with, '*Le Dieu était là.*'

I have quoted this extract from Sarcey's criticism, published on the 7th June 1880, at length, not only because it is interesting in itself, and

[1] *Quarante Ans de Théâtre*, vol. vi, p. 223.

valuable historically, but because it provides us with an example of what among English critics at least is rare, discrimination between two great and different artists: in England the older artist is generally sacrificed to the newer, if the critics are young; if on the other hand the critics are old, the younger artist is not admitted to be able to hold a candle to the older, especially if the older is dead. Witness the comparisons made between Sarah Bernhardt and Eleonora Duse in the nineties, by Bernard Shaw and William Archer.

After these two performances, Monsieur Perrin sent Sarah an ambassador of peace in the shape of Got. He was, she tells us, an ill-chosen ambassador, and he made the mistake of urging her to be prudent and to provide for her old age. It may be doubted whether anyone would have proved more successful. The Comédie Française offered to let her go on her American tour, and to arrange everything on her return. Sarah refused, and set out for Brussels and Copenhagen; then, after a tour of twenty-five performances in the provinces of France, arranged hurriedly and at the last moment (the whole tour only taking twenty-eight days), she sailed for New York on 11th October 1880.

She arrived on 27th October and opened in *Adrienne Lecouvreur*. The performance was a triumphant success, as were the twenty-seven others in New York. And then, after visiting Boston, Montreal, Baltimore, Philadelphia, Chicago, Saint Louis, Cincinnati, New Orleans, Washington, and many other smaller cities, she returned to New York, where she gave a professional matinée of *La Princesse Georges* to the actors and actresses of New York, at which Salvini was present, and Mary Anderson, aged twenty-one.

In May 1881 she sailed for France, where she was met with a great welcome: 50,000 people welcomed her at Havre. She had been away seven months; she had visited fifty cities and given a hundred and fifty-six performances, of which the total receipts were 2,667,600 francs.

Three days after her arrival in Paris, Victorien Sardou read her a play he had written called *Fédora*, and that meant the beginning of a new and momentous chapter in her life.

CHAPTER V

SARAH BERNHARDT had a great many adventures during her first American tour, some of them thrilling. She was everywhere successful, except in one theatre where the scenery fell to pieces in the middle of an act. This, as might be expected, got a laugh. She was often wilfully naughty; she was besieged and sometimes worn out by reporters, admirers, advertisers, fans, maniacs, and autograph-hunters. But all these things might happen and have happened to other celebrities, and are of no great interest to the student of her artistic career. She says that the most important thing about her American career was the discipline imposed on her by her manager, Jarrett. 'That terrible Jarrett,' she says, 'with his implacable and cruel wisdom, tamed my wild nature by a constant appeal to my probity.' She describes Jarrett thus: 'He was about sixty-five or seventy, tall, with a face like King Agamemnon framed by the most beautiful silver white hair; his eyes of so pale a blue that when they were lit with anger you thought he was blind; handsome when calm, but when animated his upper lip showed his teeth and curled up in a ferocious sniff. . . . He was a terrible man, extremely intelligent, but from childhood he had had to fight the world, and he despised mankind. Although he had suffered himself a great deal, he had no pity for the sufferings of others. He always said that every man was adequately armed for self-defence. He pitied women, did not care for them, but was always ready to help them. He was very rich, very economical, but not stingy. "I made my way in life," he often said to me, "by the aid of two weapons, honesty and a revolver. In business honesty is the most terrible weapon a man can use against rascals and rogues. The former do not know what it is, and the latter do not believe in it; while a revolver is an admirable invention for forcing crooks and rogues to keep their word." '[1]

Such a man was clearly proof against all tantrums, brain-storms, follies and whims. He did not care how temperamental she was, and she liked him and respected him for it.

[1] Sarah Bernhardt, *Ma Double Vie,* vol. ii, p. 183.

SARAH BERNHARDT

Sarah Bernhardt was fundamentally sensible, and Jarrett taught her not to stifle her good sense, but to use it; this recalls to my mind one of those flashing remarks she would sometimes make. Talking of egoism, she once wrote in a book: *'L'être intelligent en fait une vertu; les imbéciles un vice.'*

Sarah Bernhardt's colleagues and the chief theatrical and literary critics of the day implored her not to leave the Comédie Française; and when she had left it, they implored her to come back. Long after she had refused to return the critics never ceased imploring her to do so. They argued thus: instead of touring the world and playing in inferior plays surrounded by an inadequate cast to audiences which are incapable of appreciating your art to the full, and often will not understand a word of what you are saying, and sometimes will go and see you as they might go and see a living skeleton or a mermaid in a tank (or *'un veau à cinq pattes'*), come back to the Théâtre Français, where you will never be asked to play in anything that is unworthy of your talent, where you will be surrounded by a cast worthy of you, where you will play to an audience which will respond to every tone and accent of your lyre, and to every shade of your intonation; and moreover, an audience which loves you and which is ready to forgive you all your faults and follies because of the great artistic treats you have afforded it.[1]

What they were really asking her to do was to be a cog in an exquisite machine, to figure in a chorus with an occasional solo; and she herself knew that she had the capacity and the vocation to be a prima donna. Also, when she was at the Théâtre Français she was bound to submit, however reluctantly, to the discipline of the house, and she was liable to be cast for parts that did not suit her, and which she knew she could do nothing with. Her instincts in these matters were infallible. Those of the managers were not. If she said she saw nothing in a part, there was nothing in it for her; and if managers disbelieved her (which they sometimes did), they found out too late and to their cost that they were wrong and she was right. Sarah Bernhardt was a genius, and genius is bound to find full self-expression and to take ist own way; it cannot possibly be confined to

[1] See Lemaître, *Les Contemporains*, vol. ii, p. 210.

a well-drilled repertory company, however perfect, to play the part of one instrument in a perfect orchestra. It must be first or nothing. And genius on the stage, to find its fullest expression, does not need the best plays; because that same genius will often distort and make hay and havoc of a masterpiece to suit its ends, and will be better served by a play which, although not a serious contribution to thought, not a true picture of manners, nor an exquisite work of art, sometimes perhaps nothing more than a scenario or a libretto (*La Dame aux Camélias,* for instance, is hardly anything more than a libretto, and would not have lived as a play three weeks had it not been, ever since its first production, through many generations, a wonderful vehicle for an actress of genius to create a masterpiece with), is nevertheless theatrically effective, and appropriate and serviceable for talent, or maybe genius, of a particular kind.

Take the case of Henry Irving. Irving played a great many Shakespearean parts, and some of them, it is said, he played very well; but they were not his greatest triumphs. He distorted, travestied, and sometimes butchered Shakespeare to make a Lyceum holiday. His Shylock dislocated the whole play and threw it out of balance, but *he* was magnificent. His Romeo was universally said to be grotesque, and yet when he stepped into the vault of the Capulets with death in his soul and despair on his face, Ellen Terry has placed on record that she nearly fainted at the sight.[1] Interesting as these achievements were, his successes were more popular and more artistically satisfactory when the occasions, instead of being Shakespeare, were plays like *The Bells,* or Wills' *Charles I,* or *The Lyons Mail,* when it did not matter what he did with the play, when the play without him was nothing, just so much material, practically a scenario of which his personality made a masterpiece—the masterpiece being his performance.

The same thing is true about Eleonora Duse. People said it was a pity she played in inferior plays, and she talked herself of an ideal theatre somewhere out-of-doors in Greece, and in the future, where she should some day act tragedies by great poets; but the fact remains that she was a failure in Shakespeare's *Antony and Cleopatra,* and not over-successful in d'Annunzio's *Paolo*

[1] *Memoirs,* p. 167.

and Francesca; and her great successes were in the plays of Sudermann, Sardou, Alexandre Dumas *fils,* Pinero and Maurice Donnay.

The same thing is to a certain extent true about Sarah Bernhardt, although there is one great reservation to be made, or rather, two reservations. She was, firstly, an exquisite speaker of verse: nobody, before or since, has ever spoken French verse more melodiously; and her voice could make any verse sound lovely —so much so that when she brought *Le Passant,* by the then unknown poet François Coppée, to the manager of the Odéon and begged him to let her read it to him, he said, and rightly: certainly not, he would read it himself: he did not trust that *voix trompeuse.*

Thus, when she found among the classical plays of the French repertory parts such as Phèdre or Andromaque, or, among those of the romantic repertory, parts such as Doña Sol or the Queen in *Ruy Blas,* these parts, being lent her instinctive interpretation and matchless voice, and being in themselves highly-wrought pieces of art, became when she repeated them, by the nature of the case, her highest artistic achievements. Secondly, if she found a part that was written by a man of genius—say Hamlet or Musset's Lorenzaccio, her instincts, which were those of a genius, seemed to respond and make incarnate the genius of the poet. Deep called to deep.

This is what Matthew Arnold called in the case of Rachel 'intellectual power'; but, as I have already said, I do not believe it was intellectual power at all, but supreme infallible theatrical instinct. The part had to suit her. Apart from *Phèdre* and *Andromaque,* she had little use for Racine. She played Monime in *Mithridate* at the Français against her will, and Sarcey said she was frankly bad in it. There was in that part, she said, not a single point (*pas un seul effet*)—nothing whatever for her. Later in her life she played Hermione in *Andromaque,* and that was not a success. She never played in Corneille at all. Her triumphs in Racine and Victor Hugo were her finest artistic triumphs, but it was not in these plays that she showed all she could do, or rather what she and nobody else could do. For great actresses had been great in Racine and Victor Hugo. Sarah was to do certain things in other parts that nobody else could ever possibly have done at all;

and the proof of this is, that when the French critics saw her play *Adrienne Lecouvreur* and *Froufrou* in London for the first time, and still more, when they saw her play *La Dame aux Camélias* for the first time in Paris after her return from America, they were unanimously agreed that in these plays she revealed facets of genius they had not dreamed were there. And yet they had all seen her play Phèdre and Doña Sol, and these parts had drawn on all the artistry and poetry that was in her, but not on all the facets of her genius, nor on all the resources of her peculiar power and personality.

Sardou was the first person to guess what undiscovered provinces were yet to be annexed to her kingdom, and he set about to write plays for her. Later on some people said that this was a misfortune, and that Sarah's artistic career was marred if not ruined by acting in machine-made plays by Sardou, when she might have been giving Shakespeare and Ibsen or discovering new French poets and playwrights.

But this did not prevent Sarah from making experiments and discoveries in the work of new authors and in the old repertory (for instance, she produced plays by Jules Lemaître, Silvestre,

Sudermann, Paul Hervieu, d'Annunzio, Catulle Mendès, Tristan Bernard, Zamaçois and Benelli, not to mention Rostand, and in the old repertory she played in Molière and revived Victor Hugo's *Angelo* and *Lucrèce Borgia*); and apart from this fact, Sarah and Providence probably knew better, namely, that she was doing her duty in that state of art to which she had been called. Many years later, when she had a theatre of her own, Marion Crawford, the novelist, wrote a play for her on the subject of Paolo and Francesca, which was performed. He told me that when he first read the scenario of the play to her, every now and then she interrupted him saying: 'That is good theatre.' (*'C'est du bon théâtre.'*) I believe that *'du bon théâtre'* was all that she looked for in any play, for she knew instinctively that it was only in plays that were theatrically effective that she could exercise her peculiar gifts. But she did not much care, when she saw the effect was there, whether the play was by Victor Hugo or F. C. Phillips (author of *As in a Looking-Glass*). In 1889 she produced a play called *Léna,* drawn from that novel, and certainly as a play no greater rubbish was ever written. It gave her the opportunity of a great death-scene, which she was perhaps right in thinking one of her very greatest achievements. She looked upon plays as a bootmaker looks upon leather—is it suitable or not for making a boot? If so, well and good. If not, let us find something that is. Can I make a new kind of boot with this particular leather? If so, well and good. But she was a bold and adventurous bootmaker, and ready for any experiment in the oldest or newest leather.

Now, of all theatrically effective playwrights, Sardou is one of the most theatrically effective that have ever lived. Above all things, amusing (an *amuseur*), never a bore, and in addition to his, consummately clever in preparing his effects, in prolonging and exciting the suspense of an audience, and, further, when he chose, of thrilling an audience; moreover, intensely versatile, his powers ranging from comedy such as *A Scrap of Paper* (made so popular by the Kendals in England), historical drama such as *Patrie* and *La Haine* and *Théodora,* to scabrous farce such as *Divorçons!* political satire such as *Rabagas,* and drawing-room drama such as *Nos Intimes* (played by the Bancrofts at the Haymarket, and called *Peril*); drama such as *Dora* (*Diplomacy*) and historical comedy such as *Madame Sans-Gêne*. Sardou's plays have been played all over the world in every language, and they have never bored an audience; and it is the most undeniable and incontestable merit and asset a playwright can desire. In the nineties and nineteen-hundreds it was the fashion to despise Sardou and to talk of Sardoodledom, and to deplore his lack of the modern spirit, his absence of 'message,' his inability to grapple with sexual and political problems of the day, his want of political and ethical outlook. He was blamed for not being Ibsen, and later for not being Tchekov, but Sardou never did wish to be anything else but a playwright, writing *du bon théâtre* on interesting, amusing, moving and picturesque subjects; his only aim was to interest, amuse, move, excite and thrill the large public that went to plays; and being a man of genius, he did this as well as any playwright has ever done it; and now that the modern spirit of the nineties and nineteen-hundreds is old-fashioned, dead and forgotten, and a modern audience is more prepared to be amused by an expressionist performance of Punch and Judy, or of a transpontine melodrama, than by a play of Ibsen, who even in Denmark is totally eclipsed, modern critics would gladly accept a latter-day Sardou if there were one. The nearest approach to one has been Edgar Wallace; and an audience is still ready to applaud Sardou's plays if there is anyone able to act them. *Diplomacy,* for instance, has been successful every time it has been revived in any country. Those who blame and despise Sardou never realise how rare and consummate were his gifts; as if to write a play like Sardou's were child's play; just as when Oscar Wilde's comedies were being successful the critics said his manner of writing plays was a trick, which made Bernard Shaw exclaim he seemed to be the only man in London who was not capable of writing an Oscar Wilde play at a minute's notice.

The truth was that since Scribe nobody had displayed such ingenious stage-craft as Sardou, and no playwright since his death has equalled, still less surpassed him, in his particular province.

CHAPTER VI

When Sarah Bernhardt returned from America she started on a voyage of discovery all over Europe. She began with England, and in June 1881 she played *La Dame aux Camélias* in London, a play which up till then had been forbidden except in a mutilated and bowdlerised form by the censorship. Sarcey, in writing of this performance, which he went to London to see, said:

'Mademoiselle Sarah Bernhardt has given us in *La Dame aux Camélias* a pleasure which is a very rare thing in the theatre, an enchanting, a delicious pleasure: that of witnessing something perfect: perfect, with nothing of the correct and cold perfection which is born of negative qualities, and is in reality only an exemption from striking faults, but an animated and living perfection.'[1]

In fact, he says that he has witnessed what he had said years before, in writing of the

[1] *Quarante Ans de Théâtre*, vol. v, p. 189.

earlier efforts of the same actress, was something which he thought could never be: a blend of all the gifts in one artist: perfection. (See Chapter II, p. 21.)

Sardou, before this performance, had already divined the kind of riches that had not been revealed in Sarah Bernhardt's genius, and he set about to exploit them: to write plays which should exhibit and make use of this undiscovered wealth. *Fédora* was the first of these plays; but before it was produced at the Vaudeville Sarah Bernhardt completed her journey all over Europe, which was not without event and excitement. She nearly died at Genoa; at St. Petersburg the public went mad about her, the students took the horses from her carriage, and people paid large sums for seats; at Kiev she was insulted as a Jewess; and at Odessa she was stoned. On 4th April of the following year (1882), in London, she married an actor in her company, a Greek called Damala, and went with him to Greece; but by the time the European tour was ended and she came back to Paris in the autumn, this marriage was also at an end.

The next event of importance in her career was the production of *Fédora*. The first night was on the 12th December 1882. Pierre Berton played Ipanoff, the hero.

Fédora is a drawing-room melodrama about Russian Nihilists, who in the eighties were a safe and popular theme for such melodrama or for bedside fiction. Nihilists were then a stage asset, just as gangsters were in the year 1932. Fédora, who is a Russian princess, is, of course, no more like a Russian princess than Jules Verne's *Michael Strogoff* is like a novel of Tolstoy: but that was of little consequence. What matters is that Fédora is an extremely effective stage Russian princess. Her husband is brought home dead from a house in St. Petersburg, where he has been keeping a rendezvous, but it is thought that he has been killed by a Nihilist called Ipanoff, and Fédora decides to take her revenge on this man for the murder of her husband. She meets him in Paris, succeeds in making him fall in love with her, but falls in love with him herself during the process. And just when all her carefully-arranged plans of revenge, of having him arrested and sent to Siberia, are about to come off, she finds out that the whole story is a mare's nest: that he has nothing to do with Nihilists or with the death

SARAH BERNHARDT

of her husband, who had been unfaithful to her. She keeps him in her house to prevent his being arrested, and she takes poison before he finds out the truth.

The play is constructed with amazing cunning, especially the first scene, by its accumulation of small and pregnant detail, and the rapidity of the dialogue. Sarcey's record of the first night of this play is extraordinarily interesting. The play had raised the highest expectations, the house being sold out for weeks beforehand. It was successful from the first; but the success, says Sarcey, was first due to Sardou, and to the skilful manner with which he had administered graduated doses of suspense and expectation; and not to the acting, for, as so often happened on first nights, Sarah was overcome by stage fright, and the rest of the cast caught her nervousness and were almost inaudible. With the second act Sarah's nervousness vanished, and she startled the audience for the first time with one of those explosions of tigerish passion and feline seduction which, whether they are good art or bad, nobody has been able to match since. Sarcey sums up the play lastly by saying it is only a sensational paragraph ('*un fait divers*') cut up into slices by a prodigiously skilful hand and executed with an incomparable brio of dialogue; and, while paying the warmest tribute to Sarah Bernhardt's power, he records for the first time the absence of her golden sing-song, which he says was no longer heard in this part.

But it is when one sees this play acted by anyone else that the scale and magnitude and quality of Sarah's genius become evident. I have seen the play badly acted by others, when it was null, and I have seen it acted by Eleonora Duse, and her performance brought to light not only the peculiar quality of Sarah's genius, but also the subtle skill of Victorien Sardou in manipulating the stops of the unique instrument he was dealing with.

Writing of Duse's performance directly after I saw her, I wrote:

'The play is an ingeniously-contrived machine for eliciting certain electrical effects from Sarah Bernhardt, and when we witness that process we are convinced that that process is a thrilling one. But in order to elicit Madame Duse's effects the machine would have to be constructed on a different plan. *Fédora* is just what is *not* needed for Madame Duse. She tries to make Fédora a convincingly natural and real woman, but we are not convinced. The truth is, we do not want to be convinced that Fédora is a real person, and that this wild and lurid sequence of improbabilities and absurdities is a page snatched out of life.

'We wish, in going to a melodrama, to be thrilled, to feel an electric shock. We miss in Madame Duse's performance the electricity; and never, in spite of her gallant efforts and her consummate technique, do we get the impression which she nearly always gives us, that we are really present, that what we see is real. It is not her fault, it is the fault of the play, which must be accepted and acted as a melodrama or not at all.

'Unfortunately it was made like a tight-fitting garment for Sarah Bernhardt, and we have never seen another artist who could wear it.' [1]

The proof of the pudding is in the eating of it. Sarah could fill a theatre in any country of the globe when she played Fédora. Duse, in the same part, could not.

In the summer of the following year, 1883,

[1] *Morning Post,* 10th July 1905.

she played in *Fédora* in London, and triumphed in it. Later on in the year she migrated to the Porte Saint-Martin, where she played in *La Dame aux Camélias, Nana Sahib,* by Richepin, and *Macbeth*. As Lady Macbeth, in a very crude and literal prose version by Richepin, she made a sensation in Paris in the sleep-walking scene, but the performance, judging from the newspapers, found little favour in London, and she did not repeat it many times.

It is about this time (I cannot check the actual date) that Sarah Bernhardt thought she would like to play Lady Macbeth in English, a language which she never possessed and of which she could never succeed in mastering the rudiments. She engaged a lady whom I knew to teach her English: a Dutch lady who lived at Versailles, Madame de Guythères. Madame de Guythères told me that she gave Sarah one lesson. She was an enthusiastic and painstaking pupil, and she said she was bent on astonishing the English; but, when she arrived to give her a second lesson, one of Sarah's periodical bankruptcies had happened, and she was selling her furniture and starting for America. This was not the last time Sarah attempted to learn Eng-

SARAH BERNHARDT

lish. When I stayed with her at Belle-Ile in 1901 she was studying a Shakespeare part in English; I am not sure it was not Romeo.

In the summer of 1884, she toured round Europe, and on the 26th of December she appeared in Sardou's next great manifestation, *Théodora*.

Théodora is another tight-fitting garment made for Sarah Bernhardt. This time Sardou went further. He took a broader brush and dipped it in the hues of historic convulsion. He chose Byzantium at the epoch of the decadent Roman Empire: a glittering background. It was as if he had said to himself: 'I have drawn stops from my Sarah instrument you were not aware of: wait and see, there are plenty more, and this time I will ring the changes on a whole series of new stops and stun you with the gamut, the compass and the diapason of the instrument.'

Thus it was he showed us Sarah as a proud and listless Empress giving audience to her subjects with majestic languor; then visting incognita, with the crudest familiarity and freedom, a gypsy friend of her youth in the slums (for she was born and bred in a circus herself) so as to obtain a love philtre to regain for herself the affections of her indifferent Emperor husband. After that we see her making love, once more incognita, with the accents of youth and innocence, to a young lover, Andréas, who has no idea who she really is, and adores her under another name, but is himself engaged in a conspiracy against the Emperor. He, with other bright spirits, is plotting to kill the Emperor and to save the Empire. The plot is to come off that very night. Théodora, from what he says, guesses that something is afoot, but learns nothing of the appointed date or who the conspirators are. In the next scene she faces the Emperor. They quarrel, and the mud at the base of each of their natures rises to the surface, for the origin of each was equally low, and they abuse each other like two bargees (and this scene is not only good drama, but is true to life). Théodora taunts her husband with the inefficiency of his police. She tells him there is a plot on foot and he knows nothing about it: she not knowing that her lover is implicated in the plot. The Emperor is frightened and takes steps. Two of the conspirators get into the Palace. They are expected. One is knocked down as he enters the room in the dark, and as he falls he cries out: 'Help, Andréas!'—the name of Théodora's lover. This is of course a surprise to her; and, realising the situation, she throws herself against the door to prevent her lover coming in and to allow him to escape.

That was one of the greatest moments of her acting in her whole career, and the effect of it is visible even in a photograph.

In the meantime the conspirator who has been caught and stunned regains consciousness and is interrogated. He refuses to speak, and he is told in detail the tortures he will have to endure if he insists in keeping silence. Théodora is afraid of his speaking, and asks leave to interrogate him herself. They leave her alone with him. She whispers the situation to him. She tells him he is bound to give way under torture: nobody has not given way. He then says there is nothing to be done but for her to kill him. 'How can I kill you?' she asks. 'What with?' 'With that long spiky pin in your hair,' he says.

'It is of no use, it is gold,' she answers. 'But

if you pierce my heart,' he says. But she cannot do it in cold blood. She hesitates in an agony of indecision. At last he threatens to cry out Andréas' name if she refuses, and he actually does cry out the name until she stifles the sound of it with one hand, while she pierces his heart with her golden pin.

'All that,' said Sarcey, in his criticism of the play, 'is fantastically improbable, but the effect is none the less prodigious.' [1] The play moves on through a series of *tableaux* to the discovery by Andréas of Théodora's identity, and to his death, of which she is the unconscious agent, and to her finally being led away by the executioner with a noose round her neck.

Théodora was played for two hundred nights in Paris, two hundred nights in England, and two hundred nights in Belgium.

In December 1885 she revived Victor Hugo's *Marion Delorme,* and in February 1886 she played Ophelia in *Hamlet.* Neither performance was particularly successful. In April 1886 she started for a tour in North and South America, which lasted thirteen months, and during which she acted in Brazil, Mexico, Chili,

[1] *Quarante Ans de Théâtre.*

Canada, and the United States, and she came back to England in May 1887, and played in Scotland and Ireland.

These tours in America, especially in South America, were tremendous affairs. The public in South America went wild over her. They would throw their jewels on to the stage and their handkerchiefs into the streets for her to walk on, so that she should not tread the Argentine dust. Someone gave her an estate of thirteen thousand acres. All this time the legend increased in kind and in degree. The tales of her eccentricities and occasional tantrums became more frequent, more widespread and more fantastic. There was a story current that she had horse-whipped a member of her company: all that is of no importance.

But what is more important, during all these years and all this travel, her fame as an artist increased; for eight years now she had tasted of that fame that is only vouchsafed to the very great; what Jules Lemaître called in talking of her, 'La gloire énorme, concrète, enivrante, affolante, la gloire des conquérants et des césars. On lui a fait, et dans tous les pays, des réceptions *qu'on ne fait point aux rois. Elle a eu ce que n'auront jamais les princes de la pensée.'* [1]

It is a marvel that in spite of this intoxicating cosmic applause she remained sensible and kept her balance. But Jules Lemaître perhaps finds the explanation: he points out that the greatest star in the world has one master: the public. She has to rehearse and to obey the summons of the call-boy.

In the autumn she was back again in Paris, and on the 24th November 1887 she produced in Paris a drama which was the climax of what Sardou wrote for her, namely *La Tosca*. It was the most violent of all the dramas he wrote for her, and, even now, when so many far more horrible horrors have been put on the stage by the Grand Guignol—so much so that the Grand Guignol itself, having reached full circle, has been obliged to abandon horror altogether, and go back to light comedy—even now one cannot go much further in theatrical anguish than the situation in the third act where La Tosca's lover is being interrogated in one room off the stage, while she, on the stage, is being told the nature of the interrogation, namely, that his head is

[1] *Les Contemporains,* vol. v, p. 345.

encircled with a steel vice, that three screws are being screwed into his flesh, and that this interrogation will continue in intensity until she gives away the hiding-place of her lover's friend, which is known to them both, the friend being wanted as a State criminal. I say, you cannot go further in theatrical anguish; granted, of course, that the part was acted by Sarah. Acted by anyone else (and it has not often been attempted save on the operatic stage, where the fact of the music makes an enormous attenuating difference), it does not exist. But there was not only this torture-scene in the play, there is a first act where Sarah was a miracle of seductiveness and light wit; a second act which Reynaldo Hahn chooses as one of her most subtle achievements. It needs an artist of his calibre to spot her acting in this act.

The situation is that La Tosca, a famous prima donna, is engaged to sing at an entertainment given at the Palazzo Farnese in honour of the victory of Marengo; the Italians having only at that moment received the first news of the battle, which indeed had at first been a defeat for Napoleon, until later on in the day he turned it into a victory.

'In this second act,' Reynaldo Hahn writes, 'I never ceased noticing how throughout the act Sarah keeps her place: that of a paid artist singer in a party of society folk. It is a *tour de force* to remain thus in the background in spite of the natural preponderance of her personality. Sitting on the sofa with Scarpia (the Chief of Police), how interesting she is when she indicates by the feverish haste of her speech and of her behaviour her impatience and her great longing to leave the party. The touch of *cabotinage* one is aware of through her good manners as soon as her sentiment is stirred: the perfunctoriness of her curtsey when the Queen is standing out in front of the throne: her seething impatience when the arrival of a dispatch causes further delay: all this is incomparably skilful and true to life, and helps to build up a psychological picture that is greatly true. And when the news of the defeat arrives she ends up with the exclamation: *"Ah, alors on ne chante plus!"* and she is off in a hurry.'[1] My experience is that her parts were always full of trivial details of this kind; but how few people bothered to notice them!

[1] Hahn, *La Grande Sarah,* p. 188.

SARAH BERNHARDT

When *La Tosca* was first produced, Jules Lemaître protested against the torture-scene (and indeed against the whole play). 'Once given the situation,' he writes, 'anyone could have written the scene; anyone and anyhow. What La Tosca is undergoing is so violent and so simple that it can only be expressed by screams, groans, howls and sobs; or solely by gesture, wringing of hands, tearing of hair, and knees dragged on the ground. Or simply not at all: by the motionless silence of Niobe.'[1]

All this is indeed true, but there is another point which he does not mention: if these violent situations are to be expressed, whether by screams of agony, demented gestures, or by a marble-like silence, there was only one person who could express them, and that person was Sarah Bernhardt. Nobody who ever saw her in that part could ever forget it. Nobody who saw her in that terrible third act could forget her expression when she first realises what is happening. You felt the electric touch that she meant you to think was passing through La Tosca. Nobody could ever forget the thud

[1] *Impressions de Théâtre*, vol. ii, p. 136.

of her straight full-length fall at the end of the act. It was not a question of anyone else doing it more or less well; others have not been able to do it at all.

CHAPTER VII

IN 1888, after *La Tosca* had had a long run in Paris, Sarah Bernhardt toured in France until the month of July. In July she had a season in London, where she played *La Tosca*, and for one or two nights at the end of this season *Françillon*, by Alexandre Dumas *fils*, in which Bartet had created the leading part at the Théâtre Français in Paris in January 1887, and Sarah proved that she could take high comedy in her stride. She toured in Belgium, Holland, Austria, Turkey, Egypt, Russia, Sweden and Norway, until March 1889.

My uncle, Lord Cromer, speaking of her visit to Cairo, told me that one of the Egyptian officials, Bloum Pasha, said to him after seeing her perform in *La Tosca: 'C'est chose,'* a phrase used by Turks to express something catastrophic.

In 1889 she reached the low-water mark of all the plays she ever produced when she produced a play called *Léna* (15th April 1889), an adaptation from a novel of F. C. Phillips', *As in a Looking-Glass*. It was the year of the Paris Exhibition, and I saw her play in it. The plot tells the story of Léna, who, at the bidding of a former lover turned blackmailer, is led to try and marry a Scotch peer for his money. This she accomplishes successfully; but in the process she falls in love with the Scotch peer in earnest. They are married, and safe in Scotland, when the blackmailer reappears and asks Léna for money, or he will tell. The Scotch peer has the blackmailer arrested and throws the letters given him as proofs into the fire; but left alone with Léna he tells her that he believes the blackmailer's story is true. She does not deny it; she confesses the whole story, but swears, with tears and sobs, that she really loved and really loves him.

He refuses to believe her and leaves her to herself; she makes up her mind to die. Then there followed five minutes' pantomime: she takes up a knife and rejects it; she fetches a bottle of chloral, pours out some of it into a glass, makes a wry face as she tastes it, drinks it to the dregs, and she sits down on the sofa with her husband's photograph in her hand, and she quietly drifts to death. Her husband tries to come in, but the door is locked. He forces his way into the room by the window, in an agony of grief, and forgives her. She stretches out her hand and falls back dead.

Why, it may be asked, waste so much space in so short a book about a production which is admitted to be the weakest link in the whole chain of Sarah Bernhardt's artistic career? The answer is, this weakest link perhaps contained something she knew to be one of her very strongest links: that death-scene which was a piece of pantomime she knew no one else in the world could rival. It was a thing she wanted to do; that she felt she must do; and one cannot be sorry that she did it.

It is now forty-four years since I saw that performance. I was fifteen years old at the time; and what I have written is based on a letter I wrote home at the time, and I still remember some of it vividly.

M. Hahn says in his book: *'Elle trouve elle-même que sa mort dans Léna était remarquable: c'est là qu'elle tombe sur la figure terrassée par la morphine.'*

I have no recollection of a fall to the ground;

the *Times* critic mentions a fall when she played the part in London, so either she changed the 'business,' as she sometimes did, or after forty-four years I have forgotten.

I feel one should no more regret Sarah having produced that play than one should be sorry that Duse played in Sardou's *Odette:* nobody who saw her do this and heard her say the word *viliacco* (coward) to her husband when he turns her out of the house, would dream of doing anything save thanking Heaven for the production; for into that word she put the sting of a hundred scorpions.

Nevertheless it was at this time and to a certain extent owing to the production of this play that murmurs of dissent about Sarah Bernhardt began to be heard. The French public were tired of admiring her; unless she stunned them with a new production like *La Tosca,* they ceased to take an interest in her. In the meantime Sardou's vein for writing that kind of drama, a machine for eliciting electric shocks from the actress, had reached its extreme limit; it was in fact almost exhausted. He wrote her a *Cléopâtre* (1890). It was less good as a drama than Shakespeare's, and less good as a melodrama than what he had done himself. She played in a *Jeanne d'Arc* (1890), a commonplace and cheaply patriotic play, and besides this, in her old repertory, which the French people were tired of. She had always been criticised, she had always made enemies, and always had people who disliked her acting. Hitherto they had been silenced by the majority. They now became vociferous, and their carping began to tell. How low the critical barometer of intellectual Paris had descended, as far as her favour was concerned, can be seen in the criticism of Jules Lemaître, whose appreciation both before, in 1884, and later in 1893, reached great heights of enthusiasm. This is what he wrote in 1889:

'I have lately seen *Léna*, a drama adapted from an English novel. The newspapers have told you that Madame Sarah Bernhardt is wonderful in the death-scene. It is true. Madame Sarah Bernhardt is a great realist on the stage, a realist who is not unmindful of beauty. In the rest of the play she gets on one's nerves. She intones her lines like a schoolgirl repeating her vows at her First Communion. Is this because she has got used to pouring out patter to audiences which do not understand French? I am rather inclined to believe that she has become so accustomed to express violence and to figure in the sanguinary dramas of Monsieur Sardou, and to act scenes where the actors scream and roll on the floor, where people are tortured, where they kill and are killed, that Madame Sarah Bernhardt has lost the faculty of understanding and rendering less violent sentiments, those of everyday life. She is only entirely herself when she is killing someone or dying.'[1]

Sarah was destined to prove to this critic that his last sentence, although it may have been well deserved at the time when it was written, did not hold good later, for she belied it in 1893 when she acted in a play written by him, called *Les Rois*.

The critics accused her of mannerisms, of exaggeration, of imitating herself, of scamping, of a monotonous sing-song or else a metallic harshness, or a helter-skelter patter of words, which they said was all the famous golden voice had come to be.

It is worth while noting, as the critics gener-

[1] Lemaître, *Les Contemporains*, vol. v, p. 344.

ally saw Sarah Bernhardt on first nights, that on first nights she invariably suffered from stage fright, and that in the seventies even Sarcey had noted that whenever she was nervous her teeth clenched and her voice, proceeding solely from the throat, contracted as it passed that obstacle, a particular sonority which was not agreeable, and her delivery became thick and staccato.[1] People complained now that she walked through her parts. The critics begged her to go back to the Théâtre Français. Her genius, they said, was suffering from the luggage-labels of so many world-tours. There was truth in this criticism, no doubt, and yet it was rare to see her act badly. It is said that in Russia she sometimes took no trouble at all, and yet Russia and Poland had witnessed some of her highest triumphs. It is said that South America was bad for her art, with its frenzied audiences, but these gigantic tours in Europe and the two continents of America were not matters of choice, they were matters of necessity. Sarah Bernhardt did them in order to make money, for although she was constantly making great sums of money it was being spent by others if

[1] *Quarante Ans de Théâtre*, vol. iii.

not by herself; and sometimes she would literally not have a penny.

In 1891 she went on a colossal tour to Australia. This tour lasted sixteen months. In 1892, after a London season, she made another long tour in Scandinavia, Austria and Roumania, followed by South America, Rio, Buenos Ayres, and Montevideo.

She came back to Paris in March 1893, and bought the Theatre of the Renaissance. She evidently felt by instinct now that if she took a theatre in Paris the Parisian public would not be satisfied with the same old thing. She must turn over a new leaf. And she did. She opened with a serious Ruritanian play called *Les Rois*, by Jules Lemaître. It was not a great success, but it was a beautifully written play, subtle in intention and perfect in style, and the critics said that the old Sarah of the seventies had come to life again. They were destined to repeat that remark many times before she died.

In 1893 she won the universal and unstinted praise of all the most critical playgoers of Paris by a performance of *Phèdre*. Sarcey, who had seen her play the part at the height of her glory and in the prime of her youth, and who went to the performance full of suspicion, disbelieving and sceptical of the enthusiasm of those who had seen her play the part not long before at a charity matinée, has put on record that Sarah in 1893 in this part was superior to the Sarah of the seventies.

'It is strange, astounding, inexplicable, but nevertheless true that Madame Sarah Bernhardt is younger, more splendid and, let us face the fact, more beautiful than she has ever been, of a more artistic beauty, which gives one a thrill of admiration as at the sight of a beautiful statue.'[1] These were his words.

She was as poetical as ever; but she now had the authority that had been lacking then. She could play the fourth act, which she could not do before.

At the Renaissance Theatre Sarah was an imaginative and courageous manager and producer, on the look-out for new talent. Armand Silvestre wrote her a poetical Indian play called *Izéïl*. She acted in Sudermann's *Magda,* and her conception and execution of the part, although less noble than that of Madame Duse, was perhaps more true to life. Sardou wrote

[1] *Quarante Ans de Théâtre,* vol. iii, p. 230.

her another spectacular play, *Gismonda* (1894), which was more or less a re-hash of his other dramas, and gave her nothing new to do, although it contained one marvellous scene. Then she made the discovery of Edmond Rostand and produced his *Princesse Lointaine,* which was the first play that really made him talked about. This was followed by one of her greatest artistic triumphs and successes, Musset's *Lorenzaccio* (an abridged version of the original play). Many French critics thought her Lorenzaccio the finest of all her parts. Lemaître said about it that she not only acted as she knows how to act her part, 'she built it up; for now it was no longer a question of one of those *Dames aux Camélias* or *Princesses Lointaines,* which are fundamentally very simple and which she had made poignantly beautiful almost without giving them a thought and just by following her sublime instinct. In this case, she added to her natural genius for diction and to her expressive gestures a most rare and subtle intelligence.'

Here again one wonders; not that we are surprised to hear that Sarah Bernhardt was intelligent: but one wonders whether it were not once again her sublime instinct which was giving the audience the illusion of the rarest and most subtle intelligence; just as Rachel gave Matthew Arnold the illusion of great intellectual power.

Tillet wrote in the *Revue Bleue:*[1] 'The talent of Madame Bernhardt has often disturbed rather than charmed me. That is one more reason for me to repeat to-day that she has reached the sublime. I have never seen anything on the stage to equal what she has done in *Lorenzaccio*.' Monsieur Camille Mauclair

---

[1] 'Cette fois c'était le triomphe, sans restrictions et sans réserves. Je vous ai dit la semaine dernière qu'elle avait atteint et presque dépassé le sommet de l'art. Je viens de relire *Lorenzaccio*, et ç'a été une joie nouvelle, plus rassise et plus convaincue, de retrouver et d'évoquer ses intonations et ses gestes. Elle a donné la vie à ce personnage de Lorenzo, que personne n'avait osé aborder avant elle: elle a maintenu, à travers toute la pièce, ce caractère complexe et hésitant; elle en a rendu toutes les nuances avec une vérité et une profondeur singulières. Admirable d'un bout à l'autre, sans procédés et sans "déblayage," sans excès, et sans cris, elle nous a émus jusqu'au fond de l'âme, par la simplicité et la justesse de sa diction, par l'art souverain des attitudes et des gestes. Et j'insiste sur se point, elle a donné au rôle tout entier, sans faiblesse et sans arrêt, une inoubliable physionomie. Qu'elle parle ou qu'elle se taise, elle est Lorenzaccio des pieds à la tête, corps et âme; elle "vit" son personnage, et elle le fait vivre pour nous. Le talent de Mme Bernhardt m'a parfois plus inquiété que charmé. C'est une raison de plus pour que je répète aujourd'hui qu'elle a atteint le sublime. Jamais je n'ai rien vu, au théâtre, qui égalât ce qu'elle a donné dans *Lorenzaccio*.'
J. DE TILLET, *Revue Bleue*, December 1896.

speaks of 'that magnificent Lorenzaccio which was one of the marvels of her career.'

The London critics, as far as I know, did not echo that praise, but I remember W. B. Scoones, who used to prepare pupils for the Diplomatic Service, and who was half French and a keen critic of acting, telling me that it was the finest thing he had ever seen.

From 1893, when she bought the Renaissance Theatre, until 1913, Sarah Bernhardt's career broadened and shone in an Indian summer of maturity and glory. At the Renaissance, where she stayed until 1894, she produced many interesting plays, and besides those I have mentioned, Rostand's *La Samaritaine, Les Mauvais Bergers* by Octave Mirabeau, *La Ville Morte* by d'Annunzio, and *Médée* by Catulle Mendès.

In 1899 she moved to the Théâtre Sarah Bernhardt, a larger theatre of her own. She opened with *La Tosca,* and played *Phèdre,* Feuillet's *Dalila, La Samaritaine, La Dame aux Camélias,* and, still in the same year, *Hamlet,* translated for the first time into French prose by Marcel Schwob—a translation which gave the French their first inkling of what the play is about.

SARAH BERNHARDT

In 1900 this was followed by the astonishing success of Rostand's *L'Aiglon,* which marked the culminating point of the latter part of her career. It was a marvellous *tour de force* that at the age of fifty-six she could impersonate a young man in a manner which should not only be convincing but triumphant.

Sarah Bernhardt certainly made Rostand. The French intellectuals now, not only the young generation, but those who are middle-aged but yet not old enough to remember those days, wonder that anyone could ever have seen anything to admire in Rostand; and even then some of the intellectuals of the day, but not all of them, used to say that his verse was worthless (*du caoutchouc*). It is ridiculous for a foreigner to give opinions on a question of this order. But there is another side to the question on which a foreigner has just as much right to an opinion as a Frenchman. And that is the value of Rostand's qualities as a dramatist. About that there is no possible doubt. Rostand was a born playwright, and not only was his stagecraft consummate, and not only did his situations tell, and not only were they marvellously led up to, but his verse, his actual lines got across the footlights, not once and again, but the whole time, whether they were designed to draw tears, to provoke laughter, or to produce a smile or a thrill.

He may have been the worst French poet in the world for all I know, but when Sarah used to repeat the stanzas in *La Princesse Lointaine* that the troubadour made for her, and when Coquelin used to speak the speeches in *Cyrano,* and better still when Sarah herself played the part of Roxane to his Cyrano, which she did in London, when she spoke the long speeches of *La Samaritaine* and the still longer speeches in *L'Aiglon,* and when she said the line

'Père qui m'a donné les Victoires pour sœurs,'

we poor mutts used to think that Rostand was *a* poet, a 'kind of poet,' if not a great one; we knew that something was making us and the whole audience from the stalls to the gallery laugh or cry and sometimes shiver. To be just, we never thought even in our infatuation that he was one of the greatest poets, and I remember myself at the first night of *L'Aiglon* thinking in the first act, when before L'Aiglon's entrance somebody reads out three passages from

Racine, that it was rather a bold thing to do: one could not help being struck by the infinitely different and loftier plane of Racine's lines. It was like hearing a few bars of Beethoven in the middle of an Offenbach operetta. Fortunately for Rostand the lines were very badly spoken. If Sarah had said them herself they might have killed the play.

Between 1900 and 1914 she made several bold experiments, produced some interesting revivals, and achieved one or two signal triumphs. She acted a bourgeois German play, *Jane Wedeking* (1903), which, though modern, had no success; *La Sorcière* by Sardou (1903); she revived Victor Hugo's *Angelo* (1904), his *Lucrèce Borgia* (1911), and Racine's *Esther* (1904) and *Andromaque* (she played Hermione) (1903); two historical plays about the French Revolution, *Théroigne de Méricourt* by Hervieu (1902), *Varennes* by Lenôtre and Lavedan (1904); and two poetical successes, *La Vierge d'Avila* (1906) by Catulle Mendès and *Les Bouffons* by Miguel Zamaçois (1907); *Adrienne Lecouvreur* (1907), a play which she wrote herself on the theme of Scribe's play, which, however, is not very interesting save for one or two autobiographical phrases; *La Procès de Jeanne d'Arc* by Moreau (1909), one of the most striking parts of her later career; *La Beffa* by Jean Richepin and Benelli (1910), a play about Queen Elizabeth by Moreau (1912), and a play by Tristan Bernard called *Jeanne Doré* (1913), in which she reached the utmost limit of quiet and simple pathos.

The next landmark in her career was, alas! the Great War. In 1914 an old injury to her leg made it necessary for her to remain lying down and in pain. She said she would prefer to this forced and agonising inactivity, an operation. The operation meant amputation. Her leg was cut off in 1914. By 1915 she was acting again, having found parts suitable for her new physical condition and circumstance, and she played in the trenches, and in London at the Coliseum in *Les Cathédrales*. In 1920 she gave a series of special performances of Racine's *Athalie*. She was carried on to the stage in a golden palanquin. Paul Géraldy, the poet and playwright, tells me that he had not been able to get a place, and stood in the wings as Sarah went by him, and he felt that she not only looked old, but decrepit, a very old woman with chattering teeth and a withered face. But no sooner had she said the opening lines, the words,

> 'Un songe; me devrais-je inquiéter d'un songe?'

in arresting enigmatical accents of wistful and tormented wonder, than you could feel the spell binding the whole theatre; and as she said the three lines,

> 'Même elle avait encor cet éclat emprunté
> Dont elle eut soin de peindre et d'orner son visage
> Pour réparer des ans l'irréparable outrage,'

her voice became the gate of a hundred sorrows, and her eyes had in them the retrospect and the sadness of resurrected spring, and Géraldy tells me that he was ready to kneel at her feet and to cry; and the audience felt likewise.

Another play of 1920 was Louis Verneuil's *Daniel,* in which she opened in London after missing her train through a bad crossing, and having to motor from Dover.

Up to the beginning of November 1922, Sarah Bernhardt was in excellent health; she acted almost uninterruptedly throughout the winter season of 1921-1922; and it was during this season that she produced two new plays,

La Gloire, by Maurice Rostand, and in January 1922, at Brussels, *Régine Armand* by Louis Verneuil, the last time she created a part.

During the months of February and March she toured all over France with two plays by Louis Verneuil, *Daniel* and *Régine Armand.* She came back to Paris in April, and appeared at her own theatre for the last time on the 28th May. She had been acting nearly eight months at a stretch almost without interruption. In June she went to Belle-Ile, her home in Brittany, where she spent the summer. For the first time in her life she felt that Belle-Ile was too far off from Paris, and indeed I know from experience to get there was a terrible business; it meant an all day's railway journey with many changes, two hours in the steamer, and, in pre-motor days, a three hours' drive. In August she resolved to sell her property; she said good-bye to it for ever in September; it was a poignant moment for her to say good-bye to the place she had created and the only place where for thirty-five years she had enjoyed the brief holidays she allowed herself.

In November 1922 she started for a tour in Italy, which included performances at Marseilles, Genoa, Milan, Verona, Venice, Bologna, Florence, Rome and Turin. She was playing in M. Verneuil's two plays. She was travelling as usual by motor-car, but on the 17th November, as she was going from Marseilles to Genoa, her motor collided with a lorry. She was not injured, but the motor-car could no longer be used. She was now always carried about in a chair, and she had to have a motor-car especially constructed to carry this chair; so after this accident she was obliged to travel by train. This meant going to a new town every day, getting up sometimes at six o'clock in the morning for long and tiring journeys involving many changes. She finished the tour with difficulty, and returned to Paris at the end of November thoroughly tired out. It was on Wednesday, the 29th November, at Turin, that Sarah Bernhardt acted in public for the last time of her life, in *Daniel*.

No sooner had she got back to Paris than she began to rehearse at the Théâtre Edouard VII a play in four acts by Sacha Guitry called *Un Sujet de Roman,* which she was to produce with Lucien Guitry. She took part in all the rehearsals, and on the day of the dress rehearsal at five o'clock in the afternoon she arrived at the theatre to rest in her dressing-room before making up, but she felt so ill that she went home. She was suffering from uræmia. At eight o'clock the company were informed that Madame Sarah Bernhardt was too ill to act, and M. Lucien Guitry told me that when they heard this news they knew it could only mean one thing, that she would never act again. The *répétition générale* did not take place, and the first night was put off. Sarah Bernhardt's part was given to Madame Reggers, the wife of Claude Farrère, the novelist, to study and rehearse, and the play was produced later.

Sarah Bernhardt was extremely ill for three weeks, up to the beginning of January 1923, and her condition was thought to be very serious, but owing to the strength and resilience of her constitution, and to her marvellous powers of recuperation, as so many times before, the miraculous happened, and towards 15th January she began to recover, and take her meals with her family and carry on her ordinary life. In the month of February, so great was her courage and so indomitable her will, that although only half-recovered she signed a contract

SARAH BERNHARDT

with an American firm to play a small part in a moving picture called *La Voyante,* which was produced by Louis Mercanton, and in which the principal part was played by Mary Marquet.

At the beginning of March 1923 she grew worse, and it was impossible for her to leave the house, but as she could not go to the studio she had the studio brought to her. The photographs were taken in her own house, where the drawing-room on the ground floor was arranged to represent a scene in Montmartre. She was at work till Wednesday, 21st March, when she had a sudden critical relapse. So great was her vitality that on Sunday night the *Times* correspondent telegraphed to London that in the doctor's opinion there was no immediate danger, and recovery was even possible. She had inquired whether her coffin, which she had ordered years before, was in order, and had joked with the doctors. The next day, on Monday the 26th, her condition changed for the worse. She felt very ill, and she sent for a priest. The last Sacraments were administered to her in the morning; then she sank into a coma, and she died in the evening.

Directly she died her house and her household, which had hung together for so many years on her word, and on her word alone, seemed to have fallen to pieces like a pack of cards. All was disorder, chaos and confusion; the commander, and Sarah Bernhardt had more than anyone the gift of command, had gone.

She was buried at the Père La Chaise, and given a magnificent funeral. The gardens of Southern France were despoiled of all their flowers, and a partner of one of the big nursery gardens in the south of France told me that so far as floral tributes went, it was the greatest funeral they had ever known.

CHAPTER VIII

I SAID at the beginning of this book that Sarah Bernhardt's private life was unimportant; it is either too unimportant or too important for a small book; too much of a side-issue and yet too vast to deal with. Those who wish for vivid snapshots of her everyday life, acutely observed and pointedly expressed, will find them in *La Grande Sarah* by Reynaldo Hahn.[1]

Although I did not know her for a very long time, at one time I saw a great deal of her. I will, therefore, say a few words about her personal characteristics, and the impressions that I derived first-hand from my personal acquaintance with her, limited as it was.

When she died, Mr. Walkley, writing about her in *The Times,* said:

'I have spoken of her caprices, but really only by hearsay, because they were part of the famous "legend." It is, however, our duty to speak of

[1] Cp. also *Sarah Bernhardt* by Sir George Arthur, and *Life of Sarah Bernhardt* by Galet.

people as one finds them, and I am bound to say that Madame Bernhardt . . . as I knew her off the stage showed no caprice. She struck me as a sensible, shrewd, kind-hearted woman, with a keen sense of humour, and modest for all her fame.'

This seems to me to sum up the whole matter. My impressions were exactly the same.

I think Sarah Bernhardt was above all things sensible. She would quote the proverb: *'Le mieux est l'ennemi du bien.'* She knew when to leave well alone: a rare gift which she exercised in her choice of what *not* to act.

She was a good friend, a gay companion, and superlatively good company, full of spirits and an admirable mimic. Jules Huret describes her excellently.

'When she chooses,' he wrote, 'Sarah can be extraordinarily funny by the exaggeration of her similes, which always hit the mark, and by the unexpected violence of her repartee. Sarah's fun is characteristic of her strength. It is evidently an overflow of sap which is dissolved in gaiety. She hits on ideas, mimicry, answers, with a go and even with certain silences that make everybody around her laugh. She will mimic certain of her friends with incredible comic reality.'

Sarah was funny; sometimes she was funnier than she knew. She told me one day she had been invited to tea on the terrace of the House of Commons by one of the more important and intellectual of the Cabinet Ministers, Mr. Balfour, or Mr. George Wyndham. 'It was a good thing,' she said, 'that English Members of Parliament invited ladies to tea. *Cela les rend moins grossiers.*'

She was interested in people, and in the topics of the day. She was a rapid and sure judge of men and things, giving them one look-over and making up her mind at once. I remember once when she was in London she was in need of a piece of stuff to make a peplum to wear in *Phèdre,* and a woman friend and worshipper of hers searched London for a beautiful piece of stuff, and brought back to her something which looked like a silver dream. Sarah gave it one look, and said that it would look flat in the footlights, which was quite true.

She was a severe critic of acting. It took a great deal to win her admiration: she admired Salvini and Réjane, but hardly any actors and actresses on the English stage without great reservations. She told me that she thought Mrs. Patrick Campbell was quite admirable in *Pelléas and Mélisande,* especially in the last act. She admired Marie Lloyd whole-heartedly (saying she was a great genius), Arthur Roberts, Little Tich, and the English comic actors. She did not care for English Shakespearean productions, but she admired the scenery. She liked good, 'straight,' beautiful scenery, and she had no patience with the kind of play that is produced in the dark. I went with her to see models of Gordon Craig's scenery for *Hamlet,* which was later produced in Moscow, and she was not interested. She merely said, 'He is showing me a lot of screens.'

It is impossible to exaggerate or to overestimate her energy. She was one of those people to whom true recreation is in reality a change of work. What Emerson said about Napoleon was true about her: she enlarged the sense of the word 'business'; and like Napoleon, she could sleep whenever and however long she wished. Nothing, when her art and profession were at stake, was too much trouble for her. She never said, 'That will do.' Still less, 'That will have to do.' She was a whole-hearted, single-minded, very conscientious as well as indefatigable worker. Once a member of her company committed suicide during the performance, and she said: *'On ne se tue pas avant de jouer.'*

I entirely agree with what Mr. Walkley says about her modesty. She took for granted that she was the greatest actress in the world, just as Queen Victoria took it for granted that she was Queen of England. She took it for granted, and passed on. She was modest in spite of her fame, and the Barnum-like advertisement that surrounded her very name and her every act. She rose above that advertisement and all the publicity. She was simple, in spite of the complex manifestation of her art and her personality. I have thought, perhaps wrongly, that when she makes Adrienne Lecouvreur, in the play which she wrote herself on that subject, say: *'Dieu m'a créée pour l'amour, l'amour sensible, dévoué, caché, confiant et sans volonté. Oui, c'est ainsi que je comprendrais l'amour. Et je suis au contraire, grâce à ma carrière, vouée à l'amour public que je fais naître par mon jeu de l'amour: j'attire à moi les déséqui-*

librés et les fous'—she is consciously or unconsciously making a personal confession, as she certainly is when she talks of her present, which is *'tissu de gloire.'* The legend, of course, is different. My experience is that people, when you know them, are singularly unlike the legend that surrounds them; and the more notorious or famous they are, the greater the legend, the wider is the gulf between it and the reality. But according to all accounts, the elements in Sarah, as in all of us, were mixed. She, like everyone else, was a mass of contradictions; I can testify myself that she could be superbly generous, and yet insanely jealous of some quite inferior artist, who, she would say, was trying to imitate her and to steal her thunder: as if the idea were not too ludicrous.

The curious thing is that she was not jealous of other great artists, of those who might be considered her equals, but only of her inferiors. She was not jealous of Eleonora Duse or of Réjane, but of some actress whose name would be now quite forgotten.

According to all accounts, she was a blend and a paradox: unscrupulous and honest; and

SARAH BERNHARDT

in spite of a capacity for breaking faith (people sometimes complained of her *mauvaise foi,* and Catulle Mendès called her *'la grande faucheuse des illusions'*), in spite on occasions of cheerfully harbouring hatred, malice and all uncharitableness, a generous rival, a loyal friend, and a good sort.

And now, as I draw to the end of this short and extremely inadequate sketch of Sarah Bernhardt's career, I look back and see a series of visions. They reach right back to the old golden haze of childhood, as I first saw her at a matinée of *Hernani* in 1881, when she was playing with Damala: then seven years later, in 1888, I have a vivid recollection of her caressing voice in the first act of *La Tosca,* and the look that came over her face when she caught sight of the knife on the supper-table in the fourth act, and you saw the idea coming to her that the only thing for her to do was to kill Scarpia. Other visions and pictures arise: Théodora walking on like one of Burne-Jones' dreams come to life amidst the splendours of Byzantium—

'Tenendo un giglio nelle ceree dita';

SARAH BERNHARDT

La Princesse Lointaine crowned with silver lilies, sumptuous and sad like one of Swinburne's early poems; Izéïl, like one of Baudelaire's exotic sonnets incarnate,

> 'Avec ses vêtements ondoyants et nacrés';

La Samaritaine evoking the spices, the fire and vehemence of the Song of Solomon; Gismonda with orchids and hortensia in her hair, amidst the jewelled glow of the Middle Ages against the background of the Acropolis. 'Eliminate' (I am quoting my own words written some time before she died) 'these things, and you eliminate one of the sources of inspiration of modern art. You take away something from d'Annunzio's poetry, from Maeterlinck's prose, from Moreau's pictures; you destroy one of the mainsprings of Rostand's work; you annihilate some of the colours of modern painting, and you stifle some of the notes of modern music (Fauré and Hahn), for in all these you can trace in various degrees the subtle and unconscious influence of Sarah Bernhardt.'

What a pity, people used to say, that she left the Théâtre Français; what a pity that she acted in so many of those machine-made plays. But had she not left the Théâtre Français we should not have known of these things which I have just mentioned. And as to her choice of plays, we must remember that plays by new, young or exotic authors do not always pay, and that actresses must live; that Sarah Bernhardt, in spite of the immense sums she made at various times, was more than once bankrupt and often in immediate need of ready money, and not seldom pledged to play in plays that tired her, and to act separate scenes at big London music-halls, or to tour in the provinces and in Germany, which she had always refused to do, in order to have enough money to live upon. Considering all things, she was a remarkably adventurous pioneer, and when she had her own theatre, the Théâtre Sarah Bernhardt, besides the many experiments she made, she used to give a regular series of classical matinées. On the whole, she was herself probably the best judge of her career.

What was the secret of her art, and what were the main characteristics of her genius?

I believe her to have been guided by an infallible instinct, and whatever she said or whatever she did, she could not go wrong. It is impossible to analyse and define the effect of genius, but in the case of Sarah Bernhardt, there are three main factors: gesture and gait, voice, and facial expression. Nobody ever moved better. A Frenchman, Jules Renard, describing her walking down a spiral staircase in an hotel at Marseilles, said that as she came down the steps the staircase seemed to turn, and she to be motionless. ('*Quand elle descend l'escalier en escargot de l'hôtel, il semble qu'elle reste immobile et que l'escalier tourne autour d'elle.*')

No such movement and gestures, no such plastic rhythm, has been seen on the stage since then until Lady Diana Manners as the Madonna, in Reinhardt's *Miracle*—

'Steep'd in the candles' glory palely shrin'd'

dawned into life against the dim pillar of the cathedral, raised her white arms, and took off her high crown, and slowly descended from her pillar and walked in beauty; then once more as with Sarah when she was young,

'On croyait voir une âme à travers une perle.'

Sarah Bernhardt's gestures in *Phèdre* had the beauty of Greek verse. But all was so simple and inevitable and easy, so swiftly accomplished, that you never had time to think of the *how*, nor was your sense sharp enough, however carefully you watched, to detect the divine conjury.

Then there was her voice, that languishing voice, so soft, so melting, so perfectly in tune and in time, with so sure a rhythm, and so perfectly clean-cut that one never lost a syllable, even when the words seemed to float from her lips like a sigh. And in a long period of prose or verse she followed the curve of the rhythm without ever breaking it, so that 'she varied with invariable law.' In the seventies, in her first triumphs in Victor Hugo's poetical drama, Théodore de Banville, one of the greatest masters of rhyme and rhythm that ever lived, said one day to Sarcey the critic, 'You cannot praise her for knowing how to say verse, she is the Muse of poetry incarnate. Neither intelligence nor art has anything to do with the matter; she is guided by secret instinct. She recites verse as the nightingale sings, as the wind sighs, as the water complains, as Lamartine used in old days to write verse.'[1]

Matthew Arnold said that when Wordsworth

[1] *La Comédie Française.*

and Byron were really inspired Nature took the pen from their hands and wrote for them. It was Nature who taught Sarah how to say verse. She could turn dross into gold, and commonplace verse sounded divine when it came from her lips. When the verse was good she seemed to enlarge rather than interpret the masterpieces of genius.

This is all the more remarkable because by nature she had a weak voice, yet she succeeded by self-training, practice, management and tact in achieving so great a mastery of modulation, pitch, tone and rhythm, that she could express anything, from the fury of the whirlwind to the sigh of a sleepy stream. As she poured out a cup of coffee in one play she said, '*Du sucre, deux morceaux?*' and all the charm of all the Muses seemed to be flowering in the four words of that banal breakfast question. When as Cleopatra she approached Antony saying, '*Je suis la reine d'Égypte,*' one said to oneself: 'Poor Antony!' The fate of Empires, the dominion of the world, the lordship of Rome, will have small chance in the balance against five silver words and a smile; and we thought the world well lost; and we envied Antony and his ruin and his doom.

I have quoted what Sarcey says about the soft stops in her register, and it is doubtful whether (as Henry James says of his Tragic Muse) she did not express tenderness better than anything else. But in speaking of her first appearance in *Dalila* in 1873, he says that there was a moment when every one of her words fell sharp, dry and clear-cut from her trembling lips, like arrows that whistled as they cut the air;[1] and later, in writing of her in *La Dame aux Camélias*, he says that when she voiced the bitterness that Marguerite feels, her words cut like the lash of a whip. This is one of the three categories of her delivery that M. Lemaître, and after him Mr. Walkley, the *Times* critic, so often referred to.[2] Jules Lemaître describes the three manners thus:

'Sometimes she will deliver a sentence of a speech on one note, without an inflection, taking certain phrases an octave higher. The charm is then almost entirely in the extraordinary purity of the voice; it is a stream of gold

---

[1] *La Comédie Française.*
[2] See *Playhouse Impressions*, 1892.

without a touch of harshness or of dross. At other times, while remaining on the same pitch, the sorceress hammers her delivery and sharpens certain syllables on the grindstone of her teeth; the words fall one on the other like golden coins. At certain moments they fall so swiftly that you hear the noise but do not heed the sense. That is no doubt a fault, that my *parti pris* of ecstasy must not prevent my acknowledging. But often too, the pure and monotonous diction as of a wearied idol who is too aloof and indifferent to heed ordinary mortals, has something exalted and fascinating, and this delivery suited the more quiet scenes of *Fédora*' (here he disagrees with Sarcey, who says it was entirely absent in the part; but it is true Lemaître was talking of a revival two years after the first performance of *Fédora*).[1]

In August 1877, Sarcey,[2] in writing of her performance in Racine's *Andromaque*, describes the effect of her diction on the public:

'There was no searching after effect, nothing time-taking, and yet what a multitude of shades indicated by the way, as it were, and by a simple

---

[1] Lemaître, *Les Contemporains*, vol. ii.
[2] *Quarante Ans de Théâtre*.

modulation. There was a continuous tremor in the house, which one was aware of sometimes before she had time to finish a speech, as happens sometimes to singers when the house rises at them, a murmur of admiration and pleasure, which broke the verse and interrupted the artist.'

Then there was her facial expression. No actress or actor ever made greater play with the eyes: now wistful and wondering, now like 'magic casements' opening on all that was most far away and most forlorn; now like glinting gems, hard as metal and cold as ice, and now like darts of flame, piercing you with their pointed brilliance; now blazing with fury or flooded with passion; now sad with all the sorrow of all the world; and sometimes, as when in *Le Procès de Jeanne d'Arc* she faced her judges, and spoke of *'la grande clarté,'* the sights and sounds of Paradise were reflected in her eyes and echoed in the fervour of her voice.

CHAPTER IX

I NEVER saw her play *Lorenzaccio,* which French critics are almost unanimous in regarding, after *Phèdre,* as her finest and most interesting achievement. But I assisted at the first night of her *Hamlet,* and at the historic first night of *L'Aiglon,* and I saw her play in *Phèdre* five or six times. I also heard her recite a poem of Victor Hugo's in the autumn of 1899, at the Ritz Hotel in Paris, at a charity matinée in aid of the British wounded. I described my impressions when they were still fresh: and I can only quote what I wrote then:

'It was a raw and dark November afternoon. In the drawing-room of the Ritz Hotel there was gathered together a well-dressed and singularly uninspiring crowd, depressed by the gloomy news from the front, and suffering from anticipated boredom at the thought of an entertainment in the afternoon. Sarah Bernhardt walked on to the platform dressed in furs, prepared to recite *La Chanson d'Éviradnus,* by

Victor Hugo, and an accompanist sat down before the piano to accompany the recitation with music. I remember my heart sinking. I felt that a recitation to music of a love-song in that Ritz drawing-room on that dark afternoon, before a decorous, dispirited crowd, mostly stolid Britishers, was inappropriate; I wished the whole entertainment could vanish; I felt uncomfortable, and I pitied Sarah from the bottom of my heart.

'Then Sarah opened her lips and began to speak the wonderful lyric (I quote for the pleasure of writing the words):

> "Si tu veux faisons un rêve,
> Montons sur deux palefrois;
> Tu m'emmènes, je t'enlève,
> L'oiseau chante dans les bois.
>
> Je suis ton maître et ta proie;
> Partons, c'est la fin du jour;
> Mon cheval sera la joie;
> Ton cheval sera l'amour."

The Ritz and the well-dressed crowd, and the raw November air, and the gloom of the war, the depression and the discomfort, all disappeared.

SARAH BERNHARDT

"Nous ferons toucher leurs têtes;
Les voyages sont aisés;
Nous donnerons à ces bêtes
Une avoine de baisers.

Viens! nos doux chevaux mensonges
Frappent du pied tous les deux,
Le mien au fond de mes songes
Et le tien au fond des cieux.

Un bagage est nécessaire;
Nous emporterons nos vœux,
Nos bonheurs, notre misère,
Et la fleur de tes cheveux."

We heard the champing of the steeds in an enchanted forest, the song of the calling bird, and the laughter of adventurous lovers.

"Viens, le soir brunit les chênes,
Le moineau rit; ce moqueur
Entend le doux bruit des chaînes
Que tu m'as mises au cœur.

Ce ne sera point ma faute
Si les forêts et les monts,
En nous voyant côte à côte,
Ne murmurent pas: Aimons!

Viens, sois tendre, je suis ivre,
O les verts taillis mouillés!
Ton souffle te fera suivre
De papillons révillés."

SARAH BERNHARDT

In the second line of the last stanza quoted,

"O les verts taillis mouillés!"

her voice suddenly changed its key and passed, as it were, from a minor of tenderness to an abrupt major of child-like wonder or delighted awe; it half broke into something between a sob of joy and a tearful smile; we saw the dew-drenched grasses and the gleaming thickets, and then as she said the next two lines the surprise died away in mystery and an infinite homage:

"Was it love or praise?
Speech half asleep or song half awake?"

And when further on in the poem she said,

"Allons-nous-en par l'Autriche!
Nous aurons l'aube à nos fronts;
Je serai grand, et toi riche,
Puisque nous nous aimerons,"

we heard the call of youth, the soaring of first love, the spirit of adventure, of romance, and of spring. When she came to the last stanza of all,

SARAH BERNHARDT

"Tu seras dame, et moi comte;
Viens, mon cœur s'épanouit,
Viens, nous conterons ce conte
Aux étoiles de la nuit,"

she opened wide her raised arms, and one could have sworn a girl of eighteen, "April's lady," was calling to her "lord in May."

'When she had done, a great many people in the audience were crying; the applause was deafening, and she had to say the whole poem over a second time, which she did, with the same effect on the audience.'

Her Hamlet was hotly discussed. Critics were at variance with one another on the subject. In defence of her reading of the part, she said she thought Hamlet a simple character, and one critic commented, 'Need we say more than that?' Meaning to say, the remark put her out of court. But was she really so far wrong? Is it not true that the Elizabethans in Shakespeare's day had thought Hamlet a perfectly simple character? And is it not true that the modern world, starting with Goethe and the Germans, and Coleridge, at the beginning of the nineteenth century overlaid Hamlet with metaphysics which the Elizabethans and Shakespeare himself probably never dreamed of?

SARAH BERNHARDT

Sarah played Hamlet as a boy, who tried to carry out the behest of his father's ghost to kill his murderous uncle as soon as he could after he was satisfied that that ghost was an honest ghost. It is not until the 'Murder of Gonzago' is performed before his uncle that he is sure the ghost is an honest ghost and not the devil. After the play scene he sets about to kill the king as soon as he reasonably can. But it is not so easy; although, as has been pointed out, people forget one thing. As soon as Hamlet has unmasked himself and soon afterwards killed Polonius, it is not so much a question of his killing the king as of the king killing him. The moment his stratagem of 'catching the conscience of the king' was successfully accomplished, Hamlet's life was in immediate and hourly danger. Because as soon as he realised that Hamlet *knew,* the king was certain to try and get rid of his nephew as soon as he could.

In Sarah's Hamlet you were aware that this factor and this danger had been realised; and I think she was fully justified in giving us, for a change, instead of an unhinged dreamer a practical Hamlet, who set about and got on with his business of revenge until he was hurled from event to event.

SARAH BERNHARDT

But it does not matter what she thought about the part; that was all concocted afterwards; the point was what she did with it.

A friend of mine, Auguste Bréal, an English scholar, who was the friend of Marcel Schwob, the author of this version of *Hamlet,* was present at some of the rehearsals, and he told me that once or twice Sarah Bernhardt consulted him as to the meaning of a passage. He said what he thought, and she answered in a way which showed she had completely misunderstood him and had perhaps not even listened. The process was repeated two or three times running, the misunderstanding growing deeper and wider. Then, he said, she went on to the stage and played the passage in question not only as if she had understood the words he had explained, but as if she had had access to the inner secrets of the poet's mind.

The audience, on the first night she played Hamlet in Paris, was hypercritical, and the play was received coldly until the first scene between Polonius and Hamlet. When Hamlet answers Polonius' question 'What do you read, my lord?' with his 'Words, words, words,' Sarah Bernhardt played it like this. (She was dressed and got up like the pictures of young Raphael.) Hamlet was lying on a chair reading a book. The first *'Des mots'* he spoke with an absent-minded indifference, just as anyone speaks when interrupted by a bore; in the second *'Des mots'* his answer seemed to catch his own attention; and the third *'Des mots'* was accompanied by a look, and charged with intense but fugitive intention, with a break in the intonation that clearly said: 'Yes, it is words, words, words, and everything else in the whole world is only words, words, words.' This adumbration of a hint was instantly seized by the audience, from the gallery to the stalls; and the whole house applauded. It was a fine example of the receptivity and the corporate intelligence of a French audience. Such things in my experience do not happen in England: except at football matches and fights.

Whereas most Hamlets seem isolated from the rest of the players, as if they were reciting something apart from the play and speaking to the audience, this Hamlet spoke to the other persons of the play, shared their life, their extraordinary life, however wide the spiritual gulf might be between them and him. This Hamlet was a Prince in Denmark, not in splendid isolation on the boards showing how well he could spout monologues, or that he was an interesting fellow. In this *Hamlet* there was real continuity; every scene seemed to have connection with the preceding scenes.

In the dialogue with Ophelia, 'Get thee to a nunnery,' the transition between the tenderness of 'Nymph, in thy orisons be all my sins remembered,' and the brutality of 'I have heard of your paintings too, well enough,' was made plausible by Hamlet catching sight of the king and Polonius in the arras—a piece of business recommended, I think, by Coleridge; and I believe that a Shakespearean critic now says that there was a definite stage direction to that effect which is missing.

The naturalness and progression of this scene as played by Sarah were a marvel; the desperate bitterness with which she spoke the words 'I am myself indifferent honest: but yet I could accuse me of such things that it were better my mother had not borne me: I am very proud, revengeful, ambitious.' One seemed to be overhearing Shakespeare himself in the confessional when she said that speech; and the cynicism of the final words of the scene was hammered and hissed with a withering, blighting bitterness, her voice sinking to a swift whisper, as though all the utterance of the body had been exhausted, and these words were the cry of a broken heart.

An example of what I mean by the continuity of the interpretation was when the play within the play ends, and Hamlet breaks up the entertainment by his startling behaviour. In that scene Sarah Bernhardt was like a tiger; Hamlet's glance transfixed and pierced the king, and towards the end of the play within the play he crept across the stage and climbed up on to the high raised balconied dais on the right of the stage, from which he was looking on, and stared straight into the king's face with the accusing challenge of an avenging angel. The point I want to make is this: when that scene is over, most players take the interview with Rosencrantz and Guildenstern which follows immediately after it as though nothing had happened before. Not so Sarah Bernhardt. During the whole of this interview you were made to feel that Hamlet was still trembling with excitement from what had just happened; and this not only brought out the irony of Rosencrantz' and Guildenstern's conventionality, but gave the audience the sharp sensation that they were face to face with life itself. So it was throughout her Hamlet; each scene depended on all the others; and the various moods of the Dane succeeded one another like clouds that chase one another, but belong to one sky, and not like the separate slides of a magic-lantern. The performance was natural, easy, lifelike and princely. What is perhaps the most poignant scene in the play, if it is well played, is the conversation with Horatio just before the final duel, when Hamlet says, 'If it be not to come, it will be now.' Sarah charged these words with a sense of doom, with the set courage that faces doom, and with the underlying certainty of doom in spite of courage that is there to meet it.

The first night of *L'Aiglon,* though perhaps less interesting, was a greater popular triumph. It was one of the greatest feats that have ever been achieved in the history of the stage, that a woman of her age (56) should be able to play the part at all. That she was a woman, and an old woman, when the curtain went up, after she had spoken a few lines mattered no more than the presence of footlights or paint, the canvas and cardboard of the scenery. That first night was a battle—or at least it had the makings of one, not only because the audience were naturally critical, and out to be more critical than usual, but because in that year, 1900, the Dreyfus case was raging, and plays, like everything else, had become a party question. That is to say, there was a party of Nationalists who were ready to praise or damn the play, and a party of Dreyfusards who were prepared to do the contrary to whatever the Nationalists did. Both parties were swept off their feet. Sarah conquered them in the first act. I never witnessed a more authentic triumph on the stage. I never saw before or since an audience which was prepared to be hostile so suddenly and completely vanquished. I must say they rejoiced in their defeat. After the second act there were no two opinions about Sarah: all agreed that she had excelled herself.

It was on the 17th March. All the most notable people in the literary and social world of Paris were there: Anatole France, Jules

Lemaître, Halévy, Sardou, Robert de Montesquiou, Albert Vandal, Henri Houssaye, Paul Hervieu, Coquelin, and many beautiful women. The atmosphere was tense. Sarah had a tremendous reception. When she spoke the line which occurs in the first scene,

'Je n'aime pas beaucoup que la France soit neutre'

there was a roar of applause, but this, one felt, was political rather than artistic enthusiasm. The first quiet dialogue between the Duke and the courtiers held the audience, and we felt that Sarah's calm and biting irony portended great reserves held in store; and when the scene of the history lesson followed, when Napoleon II. suddenly gives his schoolmaster, who has hitherto taught him history bowdlerised of any mention of his father, an account of the battle of Austerlitz, Sarah played with an increasing accelerando and crescendo; and when she came to the lines—

'... Il suit l'ennemi; sent qu'il l'a dans la main;
Un soir il dit au camp: "Demain!" Le lendemain,
Il dit en galopant sur le front de bandière:
"Soldats, il faut finir par un coup de tonnerre!"
Il va, tachant de gris l'état-major vermeil:

SARAH BERNHARDT

L'Armée est une mer; il attend le soleil:
Il le voit se lever du haut d'un promontoire;
Et, d'un sourire, il met ce soleil dans l'histoire!'[1]

she carried them off with a pace and intensity which went through the great theatre like an electric shock. People were crying everywhere in the audience; and I remember my neighbour saying to me in the entr'acte, that what moved him in a play or in a book was hardly ever the pathetic, but when people said or did splendid things.

The rest of the play from that moment until the end was a progression of cunningly administered thrills, which were deliriously received by a quivering audience.

When it was all over and people talked of it on the next and the following days, in drawing-rooms and in the Press, the enthusiasm began to cool down.

Another occasion when Sarah Bernhardt's acting seemed to me tremendous (and here again I am quoting what I have already written, because it is no good trying to rehash first impressions) was a performance of *La Dame aux*

---

[1] There is nothing remarkable in the verse, it was as a piece of dramatic action that the speech was effective.

Camélias: not long before the war, in fact in 1914. I had seen her play the part dozens of times during a space of twenty years, both in London and in Paris. She was not well; she was suffering from her leg, which was shortly to be amputated. The stage had to be marked out in chalk for her, showing the spots where she could stand up, for she was too unwell to stand up for more than certain given moments. I went to see her with a Russian actress who had seen her play in Russia and had not been able to endure her acting, thinking it affected and listless, and wondering what her reputation was founded on. We arrived late, after the second act, and I went behind the scenes and talked to Sarah, and told her of this Russian actress who was tone-deaf to her art. Sarah played the last three acts in so moving a manner, and the last act with such agonising poignancy and reserve, that not only was my Russian friend in tears, but the actors on the stage cried so much that their tears discoloured their faces and made runnels in their grease paint. I said I never would see her act again after that, and I did not. All the same, I regret not having seen her play *Athalie.*

SARAH BERNHARDT

But when all is said and done, Sarah's supreme achievement was her Phèdre. I have never found anybody who disagreed with this. It was in *Phèdre* that she gave the maximum of beauty and the minimum of mannerism. I was in *Phèdre* that her movements, her gestures her explosions of fury, her outbursts of passion, were most instinctively obedient to the commanding rhythm. From the moment she staggered on to the stage trembling under the load of her unconfessed passion, and sighing out the first couplets of the rhymed dialogue in accents that drew tears for the manner in which they were being spoken as well as for their intrinsic pathos, until she descended into Hades, *'par un chemin plus lent,'* the spectator witnessed the building up of a miraculous piece of architecture in time and in space, and followed the progressions, the rise, the crisis, and the tranquil close of a mysterious symphony. Moreover, a window was opened for him wide on to the enchanted land: the realm of beauty in which there are no conflicts of time and fashion. 'He saw (and I am transcribing the words I wrote soon after witnessing one of these great performances, in the nineties) he saw a woman speaking the precise, stately and musical language of the court of Louis xɪv., who, by her utterance, the plastic beauty of her attitudes and the rhythm of her movements, opened the gates of time, and beyond the veil of the seventeenth century evoked a vision of ancient Greece. Or rather, time was annihilated, seventeenth-century France and ancient Greece, Versailles and Troezen, were merged into one; he was face to face with involuntary passion and the unequal struggle between it and reluctant conscience.

'There was the unwilling prey of the goddess, "a lily on her brow with anguish moist and fever dew"; but at the sound of her voice and the music of her grief, perhaps we forgot all this, perhaps we forgot the ancient tale of Greece and Crete, we forgot Racine and Versailles; perhaps we thought only of the woman that was there before us, who surely was something more than human: was it she who plied the golden loom in the island of Aeaea and made Ulysses swerve in mid-ocean from his goal? Or she who sailed down the Cydnus and revelled with Mark Antony? Or she for whom Geoffrey Rudel sailed to Tripoli, and sang and died? Or she who haunted the vision but baffled the pencil of Leonardo da Vinci? Or she who "excelled all women in the magic of her locks," and beckoned to Faust on the Brocken? She was something of all these things, an incarnation of the spirit that, in all times and in all countries, whether she be called Lilith or Lamia or La Gioconda, in the semblance of a "Belle Dame sans Merci," bewitches the heart and binds the brain of man with a spell, and makes the world seem a dark and empty place without her, and death for her sake and in her sight a joyous thing.

'So used we to dream when we saw those harmonious gestures and heard that matchless utterance. Then the curtain fell, and we remembered that it was only a play, and that even Sarah Bernhardt must "fare as other Empresses," and "wane with enforc'd and necessary change."

'Nevertheless, we give thanks—we that have lived in her day; for, whatever the future may bring, there will never be another Sarah Bernhardt:

> Yea, they shall say, earth's womb has borne in vain
> New things, and never this best thing again.'

SARAH BERNHARDT

Thus I wrote after witnessing one of her great performances; and I remember going to see her between the acts, and finding her reading out her part, which was copied out in a copybook: murmuring the lines, and saying to herself, with tears in her eyes, '*Quel rôle! Quel rôle!*' —fearful, even then, of succumbing.

She never played *Phèdre* twice running, and during her whole career the times she played it were few and far between. A French writer, Raymond Recouly, told me that once in London he gave a lecture on *Phèdre* before one of her performances at a matinée.

The lecture was not to begin till two o'clock, and he only arrived a short time before two, thinking that Sarah Bernhardt was sure to be late. He found that she had been at the theatre since half-past twelve by herself: and when he asked her why she did this, she said that when she played *Phèdre* she always needed an hour and a half of quiet (*recueillement*) beforehand. Whenever I read the play now, amongst the crowd of visions and the sounds of that symphony which was her Phèdre, the moments I remember most vividly are, first, her look as of a hunted animal caught in a trap, when in the first act Oenone first speaks the name of **Hippolyte**, and **Phèdre** cries out, as though feeling the fangs of a steel trap close:

'C'est toi qui l'as nommé.'

Then I see her sitting rigid with horror on her golden throne as she reflects that her father is Judge in Hell, and there is no refuge for her, the guilty one, either on earth, in the sky, or under the earth:

'Minos juge aux enfers tous les pâles humains.'

As she said the line her eyes reflected the visions of Virgil and of Dante:

'Terribiles visu formae: Letumque, Labosque!'

There was a line she charged with so great a sorrow and so great a load of beauty that one thought Racine must have stirred in his tomb as she said:

'On ne voit pas deux fois le rivage des morts.'

But perhaps most beautiful of all, and as striking in its restraint as the explosions of the preceding acts were formidable in their fury, was her utterance of Phèdre's final speech:

'J'ai voulu, devant vous exposant mes remords,
Par un chemin plus lent descendre chez les morts.'

After the storm and stress, the exultations and agonies, she breathed out that final confession with a unity of tone and an absence of gesture and of facial expression which the close of a tragedy demands. She spoke, as if she were already dead, with an impersonality and aloofness, of what was no longer mortal. Her voice seemed to come from a distance, from the sunless regions, the chill of Cocytus was upon it, and as her head fell upon the shoulder of the attendant slave, the masterpieces of Greek sculpture were evoked, and all that the poets have said so briefly and so sweetly about the mowing down of beautiful flowers.

When in the future people will say, 'But you should have seen Sarah Bernhardt in the part,' the newcomers will probably shrug their shoulders and say, 'Oh, we have heard such things before.' But they will not know, nor will anybody be able to tell them, or explain to them, what Sarah Bernhardt could do with a modulated inflection, a look, a gesture, a cry, a smile, a sigh; nor the majesty, poetry and music which she could suggest by the rhythm of her movements and her attitudes: what it was like to hear her speak verse, to say words such as:

'Captive, toujours triste, importune à moi-même,'

or

'Dieu! Que ne suis-je assise à l'ombre des forêts!'

or

'Deux pigeons s'aimaient d'amour tendre,'

or

'Tout s'est éteint, flambeaux et musique de fête.'

Nobody will be able to tell them, in spite of the gramophone and the cinematograph. But those who never saw her, in looking at old photographs, will get a hint of her poignant facial expression. They will never be able to know, but she will always be one of the permanent and beautiful guesses of mankind, one of the lasting dreams of poets, one of the most magical speculations of artists, like the charm of Cleopatra, the beauty of Mary Stuart, the voice of the masters of the *bel canto,* the colours of Greek paintings and the melodies of Greek music. But it will only be a guess; because the actor's art dies almost wholly with the actor. It is short-lived, but only relatively short-lived; and nobody understood that better than Sarah Bernhardt, one of whose mottoes was: *'Tout lasse, tout casse, tout passe'* (contradicted as far as her practical conduct was concerned by her second motto, *'Quand même'*). On the loom of things the poems of Homer are only less ephemeral than a leading article, and the art of Phidias is, after all, as perishable as the sketches of a 'lightning music-hall artist.'

> 'Le temps passe, tout meurt. Le marbre même s'use.
> Agrigente n'est plus qu'une ombre et Syracuse
> Dort sous le bleu linceul de son ciel indulgent.'

The most enduring monuments, the most astounding miracles of beauty, achieved by the art and craft of man, are but as flotsam drifting for a little upon the stream of time: and with it now there is a strange russet leaf, the name of Sarah Bernhardt.[1]

[1] I wrote these last paragraphs on receiving the news of her death in 1923.

APPENDIX

LIST OF THE PRINCIPAL PLAYS IN WHICH SARAH BERNHARDT ACTED

(The part, when possible, is indicated in brackets.)

Comédie Française

Iphigénie (Iphigénie). Racine. August 11, 1862.
Valérie (Valérie). August 24, 1862.
Les Femmes Savantes (Henriette). Molière. September 12, 1862.
L'Étourdi (Hippolyte). Molière. March 6, 1863.

Gymnase

Le Pére de la Débutante (Anita). Théodore Barrière.
Le Démon du Jeu.
Un Soufflet n'est jamais Perdu.
La Maison sans Enfants. Dumanoir.
L'Étourneau. Bayard and Laya.
Le Premier Pas. Labiche and Delacour.
Un Mari qui Lance sa Femme. Raymond Deslandes.

Porte Saint-Martin

La Biche aux Bois (Princesse Desirée).
Les Femmes Savantes (Armande). Molière.

SARAH BERNHARDT

Odéon

Le Jeu de l'Amour et du Hasard. Marivaux.
Britannicus (Junie). Racine.
Le Marquis de Villemer. Georges Sand.
François le Champi (Mariette). Georges Sand.
Athalie (Zacharie). Racine.
Le Testament de César Girodot (Hortense). Balzac.
Kean (Anna Damby). Alexandre Dumas *père*.
Le Roi Lear (Cordelia). Shakespeare.
Le Legs.
Le Drame de la rue de la Paix. Adolphe Belot. 1869.
La Gloire de Molière. Th. de Banville.
Le Passant (Zanetto). François Coppée. 1869.
Le Bâtare. Alphonse Touroude.
L'Autre. Georges Sand. September 1869.
Jean-Marie. André Theuriet. 1871.
La Baronne. C. and E. Foussier.
Mlle. Aïssé (Mlle. Aïssé). Louis Bouilhet. January 1872.
Ruy Blas (La Reine). Victor Hugo. 1872.

Comédie Française

Mlle. de Belle-Isle. Dumas *père*. 6th November 1872.
Britannicus (Junie). Racine. 14th December 1872.
Le Mariage de Figaro (Chérubin). Beaumarchais. 30th January 1873.
Dalila (La Princesse Falconieri). Octave Feuillet. 28th March 1873.
Andromaque (Andromaque). Racine. 22nd August 1873.

PHÈDRE (Aricie). Racine. 17th September 1873.
LE SPHINX. Octave Feuillet. 23rd March 1874.
L'ABSENT. Eugène Manuel.
CHEZ L'AVOCAT. Paul Ferrier. } One act. 1873.
ZAÏRE. Voltaire. 6th August 1874.
LA BELLE PAULE. Louis Denayrouse. One act. 1874.
PHÈDRE (Phèdre). Racine. 21st December 1874.
LA FILLE DE ROLAND (Berthe). Henri de Bornier. 15th February 1875.
GABRIELLE. Émile Augier. 1875.
L'ÉTRANGÈRE (Mistress Clarkson). A. Dumas *fils*. 14th February 1876.
ROME VAINCUE (Posthumia). Parodi. 27th September 1876.
HERNANI (Doña Sol). Victor Hugo. 21st November 1877.
AMPHITRYON (Alcmène). Molière. 2nd April 1878.
MITHRIDATE (Monime). Racine. 7th February 1879.
RUY BLAS (Maria de Neubourg). Victor Hugo. 4th April 1879.
L'AVENTURIÈRE (Doña Clorinde). Émile Augier. 17th April 1880.
ADRIENNE LECOUVREUR. London. 1880.
FROUFROU. London. 1880.
LES ENFANTS D'ÉDOUARD. Delavigne. London. 1880.
American Tour: LA PRINCESSE GEORGES. Dumas *fils*. New York. 1880.
LA DAME AUX CAMÉLIAS. Dumas *fils*. London. 1881.
FÉDORA. Sardou. Vaudeville, Paris. December 12, 1882.
NANA SAHIB. Richepin. Porte Saint-Martin. 1883.
MACBETH. Shakespeare. Porte Saint-Martin. 1883.
THÉODORA. Sardou. Porte Saint-Martin. 1884.

SARAH BERNHARDT

MARION DELORME. Victor Hugo. Porte Saint-Martin. December 31, 1885.
HAMLET (Ophelia). Shakespeare. Porte Saint-Martin. February 7, 1886.
American and South American Tour, lasting thirteen months. 1886.
LA TOSCA. Sardou. Porte Saint-Martin. 1887.
LA TOSCA. Sardou. Lyceum, London. 1888.
FRANÇILLON. Dumas *fils*. Lyceum, London. 1888.
European Tour: Turkey, Egypt. 1888.
LÉNA. F. C. Phillips. Variétés. 1889.
JÉANNE D'ARC. Barbier. Porte Saint-Martin. 1890.
CLÉOPÂTRE. Sardou and Moreau. Porte Saint-Martin. 1890-91 January.
PAULINE BLANCHARD.
LA DAME DE CHALANT.
Tour in Australia: PAULINE BLANCHARD. Sydney. 1891.
Tour in Europe and South America. 1892.

THÉÂTRE DE LA RENAISSANCE

Management of Madame Sarah Bernhardt from November 1893 to January 1899.

1893. LES ROIS. Jules Lemaître. 5th November.
PHÈDRE. Racine.
LA DAME AUX CAMÉLIAS. A. Dumas *fils*.
IZÉÏL. Armand Silvestre. With Lucien Guitry.
FÉDORA (Revival). Victorien Sardou. (With Guitry.)
LA FEMME DE CLAUDE. A. Dumas *fils*.
1894. GISMONDA. Victorien Sardou. (With De Max and Guitry.)

154

AMPHITRYON. Molière.
MAGDA. Sudermann.
JEAN-MARIE. Theuriet.
LA PRINCESSE LOINTAINE. E. Rostand.
LORENZACCIO. Adapted from Musset by Dartois.
SPIRITISME. Victorien Sardou. (With Abel Deval.)
LA TOSCA (Revival). Victorien Sardou. (With Abel Deval as Scarpia.)
LA SAMARITAINE. E. Rostand.
LES MAUVAIS BERGERS. Octave Mirbeau.
LA VILLE MORTE. Gabriele d'Annunzio.
LYSIANE. Romain Coolus.
MÉDÉE. Catulle Mendès.

THÉÂTRE SARAH BERNHARDT

Management of Madame Sarah Bernhardt from January 1899 to March 1923.

1899. LA TOSCA (Revival). Victorien Sardou.
PHÈDRE. Racine.
DALILA. Octave Feuillet.
LA SAMARITAINE. Edmond Rostand.
LA DAME AUX CAMÉLIAS. A. Dumas *fils*.
HAMLET. Translated by Marcel Schwob.
1900. L'AIGLON. Edmond Rostand.
1901. CYRANO DE BERGERAC. (Roxane.) London.
1902. THÉODORA (Revival). Victorien Sardou.
LA FEMME DE CLAUDE. A. Dumas *fils*.
JEAN-MARIE. Theuriet.
MAGDA. Sudermann.
PHÈDRE. Racine.

1902. LA SAMARITAINE. Edmond Rostand.
FRANCESCA DA RIMINI. Marion Crawford.
FÉDORA (Revival). Victorien Sardou.
THÉROIGNE DE MÉRICOURT. Paul Hervieu.
1903. ANDROMAQUE (Hermione). Racine.
WERTHER. Pierre Decourcelle.
LA LÉGENDE DU CŒUR. Jean Aicart.
JANE WEDEKING.
LA SORCIÈRE. Victorien Sardou.
1904. LE FESTIN DE LA MORT. Marquis de Castellanne.
BOHEMOS. Miguel Zamaçois.
VARENNES. Lenôtre and Lavedan.
ANGELO. Victor Hugo.
ESTHER. Racine.
1905. PELLÉAS ET MÉLISANDE. Maeterlinck. (London, with Mrs. Patrick Campbell.)
1906. LA VIERGE D'AVILA. Catulle Mendès.
1907. LES BOUFFONS. Miguel Zamaçois.
ADRIENNE LECOUVREUR. Sarah Bernhardt.
LA BELLE AU BOIS DORMANT. Jean Richepin and Henri Cain.
1908. CLÉONICE. Michel Carré and Bilhaud.
1909. LA FILLE DE RABENSTEIN. Paul Remon.
LE PROCÉS DE JEANNE D'ARC. Émile Moreau.
1910. LA BEFFA. Benelli and Jean Richepin.
LE BOIS SACRE. Edmond Rostand.
LA CONQUÊTE D'ATHENES. Albert du Bois.
1911. LUCRÈCE BORGIA. Victor Hugo.
1912. LA REINE ELISABETH. Émile Moreau.
LORENZACCIO. Musset and Dartois.
1913. JEANNE DORÈ. Tristan Bernard.
TOUT À COUP. de Cassagnac.

SARAH BERNHARDT

1915. LES CATHÉDRALES.
1920. ATHALIE. Racine.
DANIEL. Louis Verneuil.
1921. LA GLOIRE. Maurice Rostand.
COMMENT ON ÉCRIT L'HISTOIRE. Sacha Guitry.
1922. REGINE ARMAND. Louis Verneuil.

INDEX

Abbey, Mr., 45
Adrienne Lecouvreur (Scribe and Legouvé), 9, 45, 50, 60, 69; (Bernhardt-Scribe), 105
Aiglon, L' (Rostand), 103, 104, 128, 138
Anderson, Mary, 60
Andromaque (Racine), 22, 68, 105, 126
Angelo (Hugo), 70, 105
Antony and Cleopatra (Shakespeare, 66
Archer, William, 59
Arnold, Matthew, 20, 34, 36, 47, 49, 68, 101, 123
As in a Looking-Glass (Phillips), 70, 91-2
Athalie (Racine), 12, 106, 142
Atta Troll (Heine), 19
Auber, M., 8
Augier (Émile), 33, 43
Aventurière, L' (Augier), 43, 45

Balfour, Mr. (Balfour, Lord), 115
Balzac, 33
Bancroft, family of, 71
Banville Théodore de, 18, 52, 123

Baretta, 33
Bartet, 91
Baudelaire, 120
Beaumarchais, 33
Beethoven, 105
Beffa, La (Richepin and Benelli), 106
Bells, The, 66
Benelli, 72
Bernard, Tristan, 70
Berton, Pierre, 76
Bouffons, Les (Zamaçois), 105
Bréal, Auguste, 134
Britanicus (Racine), 21
Burne-Jones, Sir E., 119
Byron, 124

Campbell, Mrs. Patrick, 116
Cathédrales, Les, 106
Chanson d' Éviradnus, La (Hugo), 128
Charles I. (Wills), 66
Cléopâtre (Sardou), 94
Coleridge, 132
Comédie Française, La (Sarcey), 123 n., 125 n.
Contemporains, Les (Jules Lemaître), 64 n., 86 n., 96 n.
Coppée, François, 13, 33
Coquelin, 104, 140
Coquelin brothers, 33

INDEX

Corneille, 48, 58, 68
Craig, Gordon, 116
Crawford, Marion, 70
Croizette, 22, 23, 33
Cromer, Lord, 91
Cyrano, 104

Dalila (Octave Feuillet), 22, 102, 125
Damala, 119
Dame aux Camélias, La, 45, 65, 69, 74, 80, 100, 102, 125, 141-2
Daniel (Verneuil), 107, 109
d'Annunzio, 70, 120
Dante, 147
Desclée, Aimée, 52, 53, 56, 57
Deux Pigeons, Les (La Fontaine), 8, 9
Diplomacy. See *Dora* (Sardou)
Divorçons! (Sardou), 71
Doll's House, A (Ibsen), 53
Doña Sol, 31
Donnay, Maurice, 67
Dora (Sardou), 71, 72, 73
Dreyfus case, 139
Dumas, Alexandre, *fils*, 27, 33, 67
du Maurier, 35
Duse, Eleonora, 34, 49, 59, 66, 78, 79, 94, 99, 118

Elizabethans, the, 132
Emerson, 116
Esther (Racine), 105
Étrangère, L' (Dumas *fils*), 27, 33, 41, 45

Farrère, Claude, 110
Fauré, 120
Fèbre, 33
Fédora (Sardou), 60, 75, 76, 78, 126
Feuillet, Octave, 22, 33
Fille de Roland, La, 27
France, Anatole, 139
Françillon (Dumas *fils*), 91
Franco-Prussian War, 15
Froufrou, 45, 52, 53-5, 69

Gautier, 48 n.
Géraldy (Paul), 106
Gismonda (Sardou), 100
Gloire, La (Rostand), 108
Goethe, 132
Got, 33, 59
Goujon, Jean, 19
Grande Sarah, La (Hahn), 88 n., 113
Guérard, Madame, 4
Guitry, Lucien, 109
Guythères, Madame de, 80

Hahn, Reynaldo, 88, 93, 113, 120
Haine, La (Sardou), 71
Halévy, 140
Hamlet, 84; (trans. Schwob), 102, 116, 128, 134, 135-6-7
Heine, 19
Hernani (Hugo), 29, 31, 33, 45, 119
Hervieu, Paul, 70, 140
Homer, poems of, 150

INDEX

Houssaye, Henri, 140
Hugo, Victor, 16, 30, 31, 33, 68, 70, 84, 123, 128
Huret, Jules, 114

Ibsen, 69, 72, 73
Impressions de Théâtre (Lemaître), 89
Iphigénie (Racine), 10
Irving, Henry, 49, 65-6
Izéïl (Silvestre), 99

James, Henry, 2, 13, 37, 125
Jane Wedeking, 105
Jarrett, 44, 45, 61, 62
Jean-Marie (André Theuriet), 15
Jeanne d'Arc, 95
Jeanne Doré (Tristan Bernard), 106

Kendal, family of, 71

La Fontaine, 50
Lamartine, 123
Lemaître, Jules, 69, 86, 95, 98, 125, 140
Léna, 70, 91, 95
Life of Sarah Bernhardt (Galet), 113 n.
'Little Tich,' 116
Lloyd, Marie, 116
Lorenzaccio (Musset), 100, 102, 128

Louis XIV., Court of, 144
Lucrèce Borgia (Hugo), 70, 105
Lyons Mail, The, 66

Ma Double Vie (Bernhardt), 39 n., 62 n.
Macbeth, 80
Madame Sans-Gêne (Sardou), 72
Mademoiselle de Belle-Isle (Dumas *père*), 21
Maeterlinck, 120
Magda (Sudermann), 99
Manners, Lady Diana, 122
Mariage de Figaro, Le (Beaumarchais), 21
Marion Delorme (Hugo), 84
Marquet, Mary, 111
Mars, Mlle., 36
Mauclair, Camille, 101
Mauvais Bergers, Les (Mirabeau), 102
Médée (Catulle Mendès), 102
Memoirs (Ellen Terry), 20 n., 66 n.
Mendès, Catulle, 70, 119
Mercanton, Louis, 111
Michael Strogoff (Verne), 76
Mithridate, 68
Molière, 11, 33, 70
Montesquiou, Robert de, 140
Montigny, 12
Moreau, 106, 120
Morning Post, 40
Morny, Duc de, 6

INDEX

Mounet-Sully, 29, 39
Musset, 33, 68

Nana Sahib (Richepin), 80
Napoleon III., 13, 116
Natalie, Madame, 11
Nos Intimes (Sardou), 71

Odette (Sardou), 94
Offenbach, 105
On ne badine pas avec l'amour (Musset), 22

Paolo and Francesca (d'Annunzio), 67
Pasha, Bloum, 91
Passant, Le (Coppée), 13, 15, 67
Patrie (Sardou), 71
Pelléas and Mélisande, 116
Peril. See Nos Intimes (Sardou)
Perrin, M., 23, 44, 46, 59
Phèdre (Racine), 22, 25, 31, 33, 37, 38, 45, 68, 98, 102, 115, 122, 128, 146
Phidias, art of, 150
Phillips, F. C., 70
Pinero, 67
Playhouse Impressions (Walkley), 125 n.
Poitiers, Diane de, 19
Princesse Georges, La, 45, 60
Princesse Lointaine (Rostand), 100, 104

Procès de Jeanne d'Arc, Le (Moreau), 127
Punch, 35

Quarante Ans de Théâtre (Sarcey), 18 n., 58 n., 74 n., 84 n., 97 n., 99 n., 126 n.

Rabagas (Sardou), 71
Rachel, 26, 35, 47, 48, 68, 101
Racine, 25, 31, 33, 68, 105, 144
Recouly, Raymond, 146
Reggers, Mme., 110
Régine Armand (Verneuil), 108
Regnier, 25
Réjane, 115, 118
Renard, Jules, 122
Revue Bleue, 101
Richepin, 80
Roberts, Arthur, 116
Rois, Les (Lemaître), 96, 98
Rome Vaincue (Parodi), 28
Rostand, Edmund, 70, 100, 103, 104, 105, 120
Rudel, Geoffrey, 144
Ruy Blas (Hugo), 16, 20, 30, 31, 32

Salvini, 49, 60, 115
Samaritaine, La (Rostand), 102, 104
Sand, Georges, 33
Sandeau, 33
Sarah Bernhardt (Arthur), 113 n.

INDEX

Sarcey, M., 10, 16, 17, 21, 21 n., 26, 28, 40, 53, 56, 57 n., 58, 58 n., 68, 74, 77, 84, 98, 123, 125, 126
Sardou, Victorien, 12, 60, 67, 69, 71, 72, 73, 75, 77, 78, 81, 84, 96, 140
Schwob, Marcel, 134
Scoones, W. B., 102
Scrap of Paper, A, 71
Scribe, 73
Shakespeare, 69, 132, 136
Shaw, Bernard, 59, 73
Sigour, M., Cardinal Archbishop of Paris, 5
Silvestre, Armand, 69, 99
Sorcière, La (Sardou), 105
Sphinx, Le (Feuillet), 23, 33
Standard, the, 39
Sudermann, 67, 70
Swinburne, 120

Tchekov, 72
Terry, Ellen, 66. See also *Memoirs*
Théodora (Sardou), 71, 81, 84
Théroigne de Méricourt (Hervieu), 105
Tillet, J. de, 101
Tolstoy, 76

Tosca, La (Sardou), 86, 91, 94, 102, 119

Un Sujet de Roman (Guitry), 109

Vandal, Albert, 140
Varennes (Lenôtre and Lavedan), 105
Verne, Jules, 76
Victoria, Queen, 15, 117
Vierge d'Avila, La (Mendès), 105
Ville Morte, La (D'Annunzio), 102
Vinci, Leonardo da, 145
Virgil, visions of, 147
Vitu, 49, 50
Voyante, La, 111

Walkley, Mr., 113, 117, 125
Wallace, Edgar, 73
Wilde, Oscar, 73
Wordsworth, 123
Worms, 29, 33
Wyndham, George, 115

Zaïre (Voltaire), 23
Zamaçois, 70

(¹)

DATE DUE

MAR 2 5 '85 Returned 4-12-85			

DEMCO 38-297